# THE ART AND SCIENCE OF
# LOW CARBOHYDRATE PERFORMANCE

## A Revolutionary Program to Extend Your Physical and Mental Performance Envelope

Jeff S. Volek, PhD, RD
Stephen D. Phinney, MD, PhD

The information in this book is provided to assist the reader in making informed choices about diet and exercise. This book is neither intended as a substitute for medical advice nor to replace professional athletic coaching. Before starting any diet, you should consult your personal physician.

Cover design by Brian Zimmerman

ISBN-13: 978-0-9834907-1-5

Visit us at www.artandscienceoflowcarb.com
Additional paperback copies available at www.createspace.com/3827132

# Other Books by Jeff Volek and Steve Phinney

*Men's Health TNT Diet*
Jeff Volek and Adam Campbell
Rodale Books 2008

*The New Atkins for a New You*
Eric Westman, Jeff Volek, and Stephen Phinney
Fireside/Simon & Schuster 2010

*The Art and Science of Low Carbohydrate Living*
Jeff Volek and Stephen Phinney
Beyond Obesity LLC 2011
(available at www.createspace.com/3608659)

*Above Evil – A Science Prediction Novel*
Stephen Phinney
Beyond Obesity LLC 2012
(available at www.createspace.com/3779119)

# TABLE OF CONTENTS

# ACKNOWLEDGEMENTS

The opening paragraph of our recent book "The Art and Science of Low Carbohydrate Living" discussed the ancient Chinese curse: 'may you live in interesting times.' In the intervening year, we sense even more movement towards a consensus change; whereby the clinical use of low carbohydrate diets in the management of insulin resistance may soon become mainstream. We are genuinely appreciative of the positive and constructive feedback from people who have taken the time to write us. Many of you asked specifically about exercising during a low carbohydrate diet, and several shared your personal experience with us. Your feedback inspired us to write this book. Now we say to each other "we live in *really* interesting times" because it's looking like a consensus change on the use of low carbohydrate diets for athletes may come sooner than their general use in medical care.

We are thankful for the support of the many people who encouraged us to address the role of low carbohydrate diets in sports and exercise. We appreciate the thoughtful comments on early drafts from Peter Defty, Peter Davis, Brian Kupchak, Brittanie Volk, and Cynthia Moore. A special thanks to those low carbohydrate pioneer athletes who were willing to share their personal experience for this book – Tony Ricci, Andrea Hudy, John Rutherford, Bettie Smith, Doug Berlin, David Dreyfuss, and Jay Wortman.

I (Steve Phinney) wish to thank Dr. Richard Handler who introduced me to cycling, Dr. Edward Horton who got me started in performance research, and Dr. Bruce Bistrian who taught me to regard nutrition as a science. A special thanks to my co-author and friend Jeff, with whom writing is a joy; and to Doug Bibus for his unwavering friendship and collaboration. Infinite appreciation goes to my family – to Lauren and Eric who put up with my abstruse verbal meanderings during road trips up and down Interstate 5; and to my remarkable wife Huong, without whose intellectual GPS I would be forever lost on the backroads of detail.

I (Jeff Volek) wish to thank my supportive parents who provided me many opportunities to play and compete in sports from a young age, Dr. Linc Gotchalk who coached me in the sport of powerlifting, and Dr. William Kraemer who taught me a deep appreciation for the complexity of exercise science. A special thanks to my co-author Steve, who has inspired and enriched my life beyond what I can express in words. Above all I want to thank my loving and patient wife, Ana and my two boys, who supported me in spite of the significant time this book project took away from them.

# Section 1

# THINKING
# DIFFERENT

# Chapter 1

# INTRODUCTION

*Humans Can Fly*

*"Perfection is not attainable. But if we chase perfection,*
*we can catch excellence."*
*-Vince Lombardi*

If you are completely content with your body, health, and performance on a high carbohydrate diet there is probably no reason to consider a low carbohydrate diet. If it isn't broke, don't fix it. But if you have hit a plateau, are in a rut, suffer from overtraining, have trouble recovering from your workouts, want to change your body composition, or simply

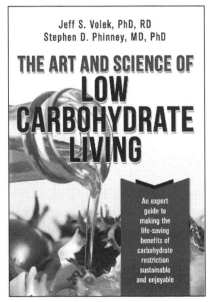

want to experiment with how your body adapts to restricting carbohydrate, then this book is for *"You"*.

*"You"* might be an elite athlete, coach, trainer, dietitian, physician or scientist. *"You"* might be a casual fitness enthusiast or wanna-be athlete. *"You"* might be new to exercise, a week-end warrior, or a veteran of the gym but aren't satisfied with your progress or feel drained. If any of these people are *"you"* then this book may have something valuable to offer.

1

In our recent book, 'The Art and Science of Low Carbohydrate Living'[1], we made a strong case for low carbohydrate diets as the preferred approach to managing insulin resistance (aka carbohydrate intolerance). However, on the continuum of insulin resistance, athletes as a group cluster on the side of insulin sensitivity. Thus most athletes do not have anywhere near the same level of carbohydrate intolerance as someone who is overweight with metabolic syndrome or diabetes.

Why then would we recommend a low carbohydrate diet for athletes? After all, the current majority group-think in sports nutrition holds that all athletes have an obligate need for carbohydrate. But despite having the best intentions, the majority view does not always represent the truth. Besides exacerbating insulin resistance, *a high carbohydrate diet also locks a person into a dependence on carbohydrate as the dominant fuel for exercise*. And every endurance athlete knows what happens to performance when their carbohydrate tank (at best holding 2000 Calories) runs dry – performance goes down in flames. It's an unfortunate reality that the human body is unable to promptly switch from carbs to fat as its predominant exercise fuel, so once the former is gone, you can't power your performance with fat (even though a carbohydrate-depleted body still has tens of thousands of fat Calories on hand).

The key fact underlying this book is that you can train your body to burn fat by simply changing your diet over a period of a few weeks, thereby turning blood sugar and glycogen into secondary fuels. Once you make this transition, you can then train harder, perform longer, and recover faster. So the simple answer to why we endorse a low carbohydrate lifestyle for athletes is that this strategy has worked for us and many people we know. More importantly, we have both conducted and published human research that supports this approach, adding to a growing body of literature that now points to the merits of reducing dietary carbohydrates to optimize fat metabolism. We have thus accumulated a unique knowledge base that we want to share so you too may experience it for yourself.

• • •

Do we understand that exercising without carbs is heresy? Absolutely, but think about it from this perspective. Before December 17, 1903, about 99% of the population thought that humans could never fly. Not long after that, the proportions for and against the possibility of human flight were reversed. In the 6000 years since small pockets of humanity first developed agricultural carbohydrates, most of us have come to believe that agricultural carbohydrates are necessary for health, and particularly for sports performance. Is this indeed true? Or is it more akin to the world view on the day before the Wright Brothers flew? Perhaps most of us are victims of Stockholm Syndrome, having emotionally adopted the distorted views of the agricultural paradigm that has us ensnared, if not enslaved.

Among scientists, and in the general population as well, some argue that dietary carbohydrates are addicting. Whether the human brain's response to carbohydrate withdrawal is characteristic of a true addiction response remains a topic of debate. However it is true that, from a functional perspective, once you light your metabolic fire with carbohydrates, it is hard to ignore the incessant signals to keep feeding it more and more carbohydrates at frequent intervals.

Another aspect of our cultural dependence on carbohydrates stems from the low cost and high per-acre production that dietary carbohydrates deliver, allowing humanity to burgeon way beyond those population levels supported by traditional hunting and herding cultures.

What is 'best for a population', however, may not be best for the individual. Elite athletes are, by definition, about as different from the general population as you can get. By whatever combination of inborn capabilities plus intense training and commitment, athletes transcend the population's norms both in physical performance and in nutrient needs. From this perspective, the correct combination of foods which best make and sustain athletic prowess must be considered as potentially unique rather than 'normal'.

Jared Diamond, the acclaimed geographer and author, notes that with the advent of agriculture in Southern Europe, the average height of the population decreased by six inches, and the average longevity declined by 10 years[2]. Similar effects were observed in Native North Americans when agriculture was adopted a thousand years before Columbus discovered they were there. Holdouts against this agricultural trend, such as those nomadic cultures (e.g., Osage, Kiowa, Blackfeet, Shoshone, Assiniboine, and Lakota) that lived almost solely on the buffalo, were 6-12 inches taller than the European settlers whose sustenance depended on wheat and corn[3]. Interestingly, the Masai in East Africa also lived as nomadic herders on a diet of meat and milk, and they too were known for their unusual height and physical prowess.

These observations support the concept that a diet consisting mostly of fat and protein can support remarkable growth, physical well-being and function – in essence, promoting the capabilities of the individual over commonly assumed societal norms.

But all of this information is old. Why write this booklet now? What has changed is that we (not just the two of us, but the greater 'we' encompassing many colleagues) are now wrapping up a remarkable decade of human research on diets lower in carbohydrate and commensurately higher in fats and protein. In the last 10 years, 'we' have discovered that:

- Low carbohydrate diets are anti-inflammatory, producing less oxidative stress during exercise and more rapid recovery between exercise sessions.

- Physiological adaptation to low carbohydrate living allows much greater reliance on body fat, not just at rest but also during exercise, meaning much less dependence on muscle glycogen and less need to reload with carbohydrates during and after exercise.

- Low carbohydrate adaptation accelerates the body's use of saturated fats for fuel, allowing a high intake of total fats (including saturates) without risk.

- At the practical level, effective training for both endurance and strength/power sports can be done by individuals adapted to carbohydrate restricted diets, with desirable changes in body composition and power-to-weight ratios.

A low carbohydrate lifestyle is not necessarily ideal for every athlete, but it is clearly desirable for some. To make an informed choice, however, every individual needs a basic understanding of how low carbohydrate diets function to support human physiology. Much of this information has been covered in our recently published book "The Art and Science of Low Carbohydrate Living". In addition, however, both the athlete and coach/trainer need to understand how to integrate this diet with training to yield superior performance, and how one can then sustain this functional peak to span a higher volume of training and competition.

The purpose of this booklet is to provide this additional information to satisfy the specific needs of individual athletes, whether your intent is competition or recreation. This goal is efficiently met by providing you with 12 concise chapters with a minimum of theory and a maximum of practical direction. After considering this information and making appropriate changes in your diet, perhaps you too will experience a paradigm shift in how you feel and function, and maybe 'catch excellence'. Humans can fly!

**Procedural Note:** We use a lot of acronyms in this book. While they are all defined when used initially, they tend to become an 'alphabet salad' in later chapters. To alleviate that problem, we have provided a glossary of terms at the end of the print version of the book, whereas in the eBook version you can recall each glossary entry by rolling the cursor over its hypertext acronym.

# Chapter 2
# METABOLISM BASICS
## A Functional Look At Fuel Use

*"We cannot solve problems by using the same kind of thinking we used when we created them."*
*-Albert Einstein*

**Snap Shot**

- Body stores of fat fuel (typically >40, 000 Calories [kcal]) vastly exceed its maximum stores of carbohydrate fuel (~2,000 kcal).

- Fueling tactics that emphasize carbohydrate-based diets and sugar-based supplements bias your metabolism towards carbohydrate while simultaneously inhibiting fat mobilization and utilization.

- This suppression of fat oxidation lasts for days after carbohydrates are consumed, not just the few hours following their digestion when insulin levels are high.

- This high carbohydrate paradigm produces unreliable results, especially during prolonged exercise when body carbohydrate stores are exhausted.

- In order to sustain a high level of performance under conditions of glycogen depletion and decreased glucose availability, cells must adapt to using fat fuels. This process is referred to as keto-adaptation which has the potential to improve human performance and recovery.

- Previously held beliefs about the magnitude of peak fat burning need to be reconsidered in the context of data obtained after keto-adaptation.

It is accepted dogma within the science of sports nutrition that carbohydrates are essential and that they are the preferred fuel for athletes. Indeed, over the last 45 years a great deal of progress has been made in understanding how to use carbohydrates to optimize the metabolic response to physical activity. This understanding in turn has driven development of nutritional approaches to prevent fatigue and improve exercise tolerance. We don't want to play down the extraordinary work of researchers who have contributed to this knowledge. However it is instructive to point out that ever since the observation over four decades ago that low muscle glycogen was associated with fatigue, most of that progress has been focused on ways to enhance glycogen levels and carbohydrate oxidation (e.g., carbohydrate loading, use of multiple sources of sugars, etc.). Little effort has been devoted to developing methods to decrease the body's dependence on carbohydrate during physical activity. The result is a billion dollar sports beverage and supplement industry that aggressively promotes rapidly absorbed sources of carbohydrate before, during, and after exercise. We contend that there's a limit to what can be achieved by consuming sugary drinks and gels in hopes of delivering optimized fuel flow, and that it is time to take a serious look at the other side of the coin.

Is the research used to support high carbohydrate diets flawed or in some way misaligned with what we know about human physiology? Not exactly – it's more a case of willful neglect. The belief that carbohydrate is the ideal fuel source and that a high carbohydrate diet is optimal for all athletes are self-reinforcing concepts that have been passed down to at least a couple generations of sport scientists. Many of the experiments conducted during that time were designed in a specific manner and data interpreted within a narrow mindset to support and confirm the high carbohydrate paradigm. The result is a classic example of conformation bias – the tendency to favor information that confirms a preconception or hypothesis regardless of whether it is true.

Despite the tenacity with which mainstream sports nutritionists defend the notion that a high carbohydrate intake is an **obligate** component of all athletes' diets, a more accurate paradigm is that carbohydrates are an obligate part of your diet only as long as you keep consuming lots of them. If you take a few weeks to break this self-perpetuating cycle, however, carbs can be reduced to an **optional** nutrient for athletes. To appreciate this alternative view, it is helpful to understand the metabolic basis of the human fuel supply.

## Fueling Exercise

Adenosine tri-phosphate (ATP) is the chemical energy that fuels body processes including muscle contraction. It's literally the energy that causes your muscle fibers to contract and produce force. At rest we are constantly breaking down and synthesizing ATP. When you exercise vigorously, ATP demands increase several-fold. Since we can't store (nor do we eat) ATP in appreciable amounts, exercise causes an immediate need to rapidly make ATP from other energy sources. The two primary fuels our bodies draw on to do this are carbohydrate and fat. How the body chooses the proportion of carbohydrate and fat to use for fuel is complex, but one factor that has a consistent and profound effect is the availability of carbohydrate. The more carbs that are available, the more carbs the body burns; while at the same time shutting down access to its much larger fuel reserve – fat.

## Carbohydrate Fuel Tank

As noted above, carbohydrate is often viewed as the preferred fuel for athletes. From a functional perspective, this is curious because carbohydrates cannot be stored in large amounts in the body. When we talk about storing and burning carbohydrate, the 'common energy currency' used by the body is glucose. Glucose can be metabolized directly to make ATP, and glucose can also be stored in modest amounts as glycogen in skeletal muscle, and to a lesser extent in liver. On average, the maximum glycogen store you can accumulate is between 400-500 grams. And since 1 gram of carbohydrate equals 4 kcal, you max out at about 1600-2000 kcal in your carbohydrate fuel tank. Each gram of glycogen is also stored with a couple grams of water. If you carry more muscle mass, are well trained, and eat a high carbohydrate diet, your glycogen stores might be increased by up to another 50% or so, but the total amount of carbohydrate available in the body is still relatively low compared to available fat stores.

## Fat Fuel Tank

Fat, or more specifically fatty acids, are stored in the body as triglycerides consisting of three fatty acids linked to a single 3 carbon glycerol. Triglycerides coalesce into fat droplets that occupy ~85% of adipose tissue cells (i.e., fat cells, aka 'adipocytes'). Unlike our limited storage of glycogen, fat cells have a vast capacity to store fat. Since fat contains 9 kcal per gram and is stored with minimal water, they are an efficient storage form of energy that can be mobilized quickly when blood insulin levels are low. Even in a very lean athlete, the total amount of energy stored as fat will typically be more than 20 times the maximum level of carbohydrate stored in the body. Thus, whereas vigorous exercise can deplete glycogen reserves in just a few **hours**, when adapted to burning primarily fat, this thin athlete has enough fat to fuel several **days** of exercise.

*Which Fuel Tank Do You Want Access To?*

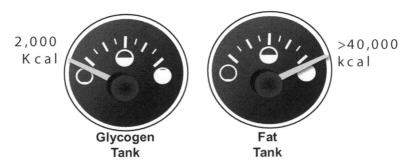

2,000 Kcal

>40,000 kcal

**Glycogen Tank**

**Fat Tank**

During prolonged exercise when body stores of carbohydrate as glycogen are depleted, there is increasing dependence on the liver to maintain blood glucose levels. This is not just to provide the exercising muscles with glucose, but also to support other normal body functions, especially the central nervous system. Decreased carbohydrate availability, particularly for the brain, marks the central event resulting in a sharp decline in physical and mental performance (i.e., hitting the wall or bonking). The current practice of carbohydrate loading increases glycogen stores and is often accompanied by ingestion of sugar-based sport drinks and gels during exercise. These carb-based fueling tactics may delay the onset of hitting the wall, but for most athletes extending beyond marathon-duration events, they will still crash and burn despite having literally many thousand Calories worth of fuel tucked away in their fat cells. Why can't this surplus of fat fuel be utilized even at a time when the body desperately needs it? Simply put, it can be accessed, but it takes a few weeks of carbohydrate restriction during which time the body becomes significantly more efficient at burning fat, a process we call keto-adaptation (discussed in the next chapter).

Keto-adaptation allows rapid mobilization and utilization of "non-carbohydrate" lipid fuel sources. As the name implies, this process involves the conversion of fat to ketones in the liver, and these ketones help supply the brain with energy when glucose levels fall. This affords even a very lean (10% body fat) athlete access to more than 40,000 kcal from body fat, rather than starting a prolonged event depending primarily on ~2000 kcal of glycogen.

## How You Burn Body Fat: Fat Breakdown

Let's take a closer look at how we tap into the fat energy stored in adipose tissue. A key step is removing the fatty acid from the glycerol backbone (aka, fat breakdown or lipolysis). This is achieved by the enzyme hormone-sensitive lipase. Although many factors *stimulate* the activity of hormone-sensitive lipase (e.g., epinephrine, norepinephrine, growth hormone, activated thyroid hormone), fat breakdown is principally controlled by the single hormone that *inhibits* its activity. That hormone is insulin. In other words, insulin is the primary gate-keeper of body fat. If your insulin levels are consistently high, fat usage is effectively blocked.

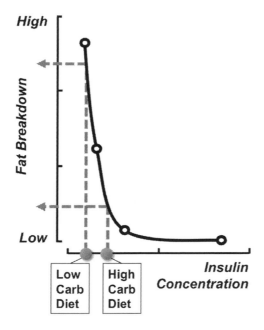

The primary nutrient that stimulates insulin is dietary carbohydrate. Some forms of carbohydrate stimulate insulin more than others. Thus, consumption of insulin-stimulating carbohydrates is a surefire way to inhibit your access to the energy stored as body fat during and after exercise.

Taking a closer look, the relationship between insulin levels and fat breakdown is not a straight line. Instead it's a steep curve, which means that fat release plummets with just a modest rise in insulin such as those stimulated by most sports beverages. Looking at it from another perspective, near the bottom on the blood insulin range, just small decreases in insulin translate into large increases in fat breakdown and fat oxidation[4]. Thus, focusing on keeping insulin low is associated with significant changes in fat metabolism, favoring decreased storage and increased fat oxidation. In case you're wondering, insulin's effect on fat breakdown does not take days or even hours, its effect is virtually immediate. Keto-adaptation, however, is not immediate. Keeping insulin low is a first step in increasing fat availability, but to maximize fat burning the body requires at least a couple weeks of uninterrupted low insulin levels (i.e., 2-3 weeks of consistently restricting dietary carbohydrates).

**Factoid:** *Like many things in life, a little bit of insulin is necessary, but more isn't necessarily better. Insulin's effects are not limited to promoting glucose uptake and suppressing fat breakdown. In addition to promoting storage of fat,insulin also potently and rapidly inhibits both blood fatty acid and total body lipid oxidation as well.*

## How You Burn Body Fat: Fat Oxidation (Burning)

Breakdown of fat (aka lipolysis) in adipose tissue and its release into the blood is only half the story. Fatty acids then need to be delivered to tissues like active muscle. Triglycerides and fatty acids are not water soluble, so in the blood, fatty acids released from fat cells are attached to a protein called albumin and delivered to muscle. Fat is taken up into muscle cells through specific transport proteins and delivered to ATP-generating organelles within the cell called mitochondria. Transport of fatty acids into the mitochondria is highly regulated, and some might argue that this is the rate limiting step in oxidizing fat. The other fate for fatty acids taken up by muscle, particularly during periods of rest, is conversion back to triglyceride within the muscle cell itself where it is stored as lipid droplets for later use.

**Factoid:** *In the well-trained athlete, muscles cells can store as much energy in fat droplets as they can store as glycogen.*

There you have it, the path of a fatty acid molecule from storage in fat cells to oxidation in muscle. But where does dietary fat fit in? Dietary fat is absorbed from your small intestine and packaged as triglycerides into a blood-bourne particle called a chylomicron. These are acted upon by fatty acid-releasing enzymes called lipoprotein lipase that reside in the capillaries that perfuse muscle and fat cells. The fatty acids released from chylomicrons can then be taken up by nearby muscle or fat cells. Once inside muscle cells, the food-derived fatty acids mix in with the fatty acids delivered from fat cells.

## Exercise Intensity and Peak Fat Oxidation

One factor that impacts the proportion of fat used as fuel is exercise intensity. In athletes consuming moderate to high carbohydrate diets, as exercise intensity increases, the proportion of energy derived from carbohydrate increases and that from fat decreases. This has been interpreted to mean that there is a specific exercise intensity where fat burning peaks, above which exercise at higher intensities increasingly depends on glucose and glycogen.

If you start exercising lightly and gradually increase the intensity while simultaneously measuring the contribution of fat and carbohydrate to energy use, you will find that the peak rate of fat burning (grams of fat oxidized per minute or per hour) occurs *on average* at about 50% of maximal oxygen consumption ($VO_2$max) if you're untrained and at 65% $VO_2$max if you're trained[5]. Exercise harder and although power output increases, the contribution of fat decreases, forcing carbohydrate to become the predominant fuel source. 65% of $VO_2$max is an intensity most endurance athletes can easily maintain for several hours. This means that if you exercise above this threshold, fat oxidation normally cannot increase to meet the greater energy demands. In fact, as you push up close to maximal oxygen capacity, there is a rather sharp decline in fat oxidation – not just its proportion, but in absolute grams per minute as well. This is an important detail that requires greater inspection because this line of reasoning is often used as justification to teach away from low carbohydrate/high-fat diets for athletes who exercise at or above 65% VO$_2$max.

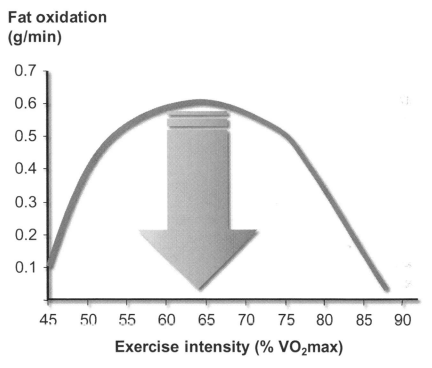

Typical fat oxidation rates as a function of increasing exercise intensity.

First, several well conducted studies over the last few decades have provided multiple clues as to why fat oxidation tends to decrease and carbohydrate becomes the predominant fuel at higher exercise intensities. It's not a simple switch that slows down fat oxidation as exercise intensity increases but rather a coordinated set of metabolic events. This metabolic symphony can play a different tune in a keto-adapted athlete, allowing significantly higher rates of peak fat oxidation at higher exercise intensities. However the minimum time for this adaptation to occur has received little attention. Most of the work in this area has involved athletes consuming low carbohydrate diets for less than two weeks. In contrast, we have published studies of 4-6 weeks duration that demonstrate a progressively increased capacity to mobilize and oxidize fat[6, 7] at the 65% threshold. Thus the time allotted for adaptation has the potential to dramatically alter the 'typical' relation between exercise intensity and fuel use.

Second, and more importantly, there is a great deal of variability between individuals consuming moderate to high carbohydrate diets (both trained and untrained) in their capacity to burn fat at rest and during exercise[8]. Studies almost always highlight average responses for a group, but given such variability between individuals, hardly anyone responds like the group average. Thus, when dealing with individuals, it's more interesting to look at the tails of the distribution (i.e., the outliers at the high and low ends of a group). For example, in a study of 300 people, peak fat oxidation ranged between 10 and 60 grams of total fat burned per hour. For some people peak fat oxidation occurred at very low exercise intensities (e.g., 25% of $VO_2$max) whereas in others it occurred up to 77% of $VO_2$max[9].

***Factoid:* :** *There are remarkable differences among individuals in both the magnitude of peak fat burning and the intensity of the exercise at which peak fat oxidation occurs.*

## How Much Fat Can Humans Burn?

An intriguing question is whether oxidizing 60 grams fat per hour (1 gram per minute, or 540 kcal of fat burned per hour) represents an absolute ceiling, or whether humans have the capacity to exceed this level? The answer, it turns out, has been hiding in plain sight for almost 30 years. Not only can this 60 gram per hour 'butter ceiling' be cracked, it can be totally splattered. Turn to the next chapter for the key to unleashing your maximal fat burning potential. The reward for many readers will be improved endurance performance as well as better control over your body composition (as in no loss of power with less total body fat).

## Side Bar - Super Fat Burning Athletes

One way to explore the upper limits of fat oxidation is to look at "Super Fat-Burners" – athletes that show accelerated fat burning and, as a result, extraordinary endurance capacity. Yes, these are animals; and yes, there are limits to their direct relevance vis-a-vis human exercise metabolism because of inherent species differences. But if nothing else, they do provide evidence for what's possible in the context of mammalian physiology. It's also interesting that these super animal athletes are characterized by an extraordinary ability to metabolize fat, not carbohydrate.

**Genetically Modified Mice.** These athletes have been referred to as "Mighty Mice" or "Super Mice" owing to their ability to perform prodigious amounts of exercise[10]. Dr. Richard Hanson and his laboratory group at Case Western Reserve University made this serendipitous discovery during experiments initially aimed at elucidating the role of PEPCK (phosphoenolpyruvate carboxykinase), a key enzyme involved in the pathway that converts non-carbohydrate substances into glucose. They created a line of mice that over-produce PEPCK specifically in skeletal muscle.

What they discovered can be described as nothing short of astonishing. These mice were easily distinguished from normal mice because they were noticeably more active, ate more food, but were nonetheless leaner. They were up to 10 times more active, sometimes exercising continuously for up to 6 hours. This incredible propensity to exercise was accompanied by a remarkable capacity to burn fat despite having less subcutaneous and visceral fat stores. These mice had high levels of stored triglycerides in their muscles and proportionately more mitochondria to burn that fat. Consistent with accelerated fat burning, these animals also showed little accumulation of lactate during exercise compared to control mice, indicating much less reliance on muscle glycogen and glucose for fuel. Dr. Hanson's observations raise the question: could there be humans with increased muscle PEPCK, or could enzyme levels be increased through a change in diet?

*Hunch:* *Keto-adaptation in humans often results in a greater desire/ drive to be physically active, likely because there is better total body fuel flow based on fatty acids and ketones. Could this be linked to increased muscle PEPCK. Any eager graduate students looking for a dissertation?*

**Racing Sled Dogs.** Equally impressive are dogs that compete in 1000 mile races like the Iditarod. Successful dogs show an unusual fatigue-resistance that develops over the course of the event that spans 8-10 days. These unique athletes are able to pull their sleds more than 100 miles per day for consecutive days in environmentally harsh conditions. The best dogs transform their metabolism in a way that avoids depletion of energy substrates and allows for rapid recovery. They actually replenish muscle glycogen over the course of consecutive days of strenuous exercise. Clearly they develop a profound ability to utilize lipid fuel such as muscle triglycerides (which shows a progressive depletion over several days of exercise) as well as circulating fatty acids and ketones. Dogs are also known to have higher albumin which gives them the capability of transporting more fatty acids in the blood, but the full details of racing sled dog's metabolic dominance remains to be elucidated. What we do know is that the dogs perform and recover better on a diet that is high in fat, moderate in protein and low in carbohydrate content[11, 12].

# Chapter 3

# A TECTONIC SHIFT
# IN THINKING

*Keto-Adaptation: The Most Efficient Path
To Accelerated Fat Burning*

**Snap Shot**

- Ketones are an important lipid-based fuel source, especially for the brain, when dietary carbohydrates are restricted.

- The process of keto-adaptation (switching over to using primarily fatty acids and ketones) can't be done 'on the fly' – it takes at least 2 weeks of preparation for this strategy to work.

- Keto-adapted athletes show marked increases in fat burning, indicating that peak rates of human fat oxidation have been significantly underestimated.

- Keto-adapted individuals can do resistance training, and show profound improvements in body composition.

Over the last four decades, carbohydrate-rich diets have been vigorously promoted to athletes based on the rationale that high carbohydrate oxidation rates are preferable to high fat oxidation rates, and therefore maintaining a high muscle glycogen level is essential to achieve optimal performance. As you might guess by now, we've just got to say, "wait a minute!" Over these same four decades, we've seen enough foot prints in the sand to lead us to the exact opposite conclusion – that a high carbohydrate diet may be neither required nor desired for many athletes. Some might characterize this as a tectonic shift in sports nutrition thinking. We just consider this to be sound reasoning and part of the scientific process.

## Why Low Carbohydrate Diets Remain a Fringe Concept

If we limit our scientific aperture to short-term studies comparing low- and high-carbohydrate diets using brief periods of intense exercise, one could credibly argue the superiority of a high carbohydrate diet. Today, however, a combination of time-tested experience and recent research data supports the conclusion that if humans are given two or more weeks to adapt to a well-formulated low carbohydrate diet, they can deliver equal or better endurance performance compared to the best high carbohydrate diet strategy. Combine this with the observational evidence of ultra-endurance athletes performing at consistently high levels using varying degrees of carbohydrate restriction to optimize fat burning, and we have to believe it is time to re-consider the optimum diet for many athletes.

Despite having made significant progress in understanding how to optimize fat oxidation in athletes, the benefits of keto-adaptation on exercise performance and recovery have yet to be fully explored in humans. There have been a number of nutritional strategies aimed at increasing fat burning during exercise such as caffeine, carnitine, ephedra, medium chain triglycerides, green tea extract, and hydroxycitric acid to name a few. Use of these supplements may mildly elevate fat burning; however, they pale in comparison to the dramatic shift that occurs after a couple of weeks of adaptation to a well formulated very low carbohydrate diet.

## Keying In on Ketones

It's important to make a good first impression, but that was not the case with ketones. These organic acids were first discovered in urine of uncontrolled diabetic patients in the latter half of the 19th century. Although a much different picture has slowly emerged over the last 100 years, elucidating an important role for ketones in human health, the negative connotation associated with their debut has been hard to shake. This is both ironic and unfortunate because dietary strategies to increase ketone production are now linked to improvements in several medical conditions, and perhaps sports performance as well. Yet there remains significant resistance to the rehabilitation of ketogenic diets, and especially their use in athletes. As one prominent scientist put it "Ketones have been Metabolism's 'Ugly Duckling'". However, thanks to ground-breaking studies on ketone metabolism, they are now "emerging as an incipient swan."[13]

When we say ketones we are referring to two 4-carbon molecules – beta-hydroxybutyrate (BOHB) and acetoacetate (AcAc). BOHB and AcAc are made in the liver from fatty acids, and chemically they retain some similarities to the fatty acids from whence they come. However, being much smaller molecules, they are water soluble, making them easier to transport in the blood (more like the simple sugars whose functions they in part replace). Even when we eat a lot of carbohydrates, ketones are naturally present in our blood at relatively low levels, but their production increases in response to decreased carbohydrate availability and accelerated rates of fatty acid delivery to the liver. This is perfectly natural and in fact represents a vital adaptation in fuel partitioning when carbohydrate intake is low or carbohydrate reserves are depleted (e.g., at the end of a marathon).

*Factoid:* *The concept of keto-adaptation – that the human body requires a few weeks to adapt to eating a low carbohydrate diet – was first voiced by a US Army surgeon and Arctic explorer, Lt. Frederick Schwatka, in the early 1880s. This historical cornerstone, lost for a century, was referenced by Dr. Phinney in his watershed 1983 study of bicycle racers adapted to an Inuit diet[6, 14].*

Keto-adaptation is a term coined by Steve Phinney in 1980 to describe the process in which human metabolism switches over to using almost exclusively fat for fuel (i.e., a combination of fat burned directly and as ketones derived from fat). While well studied and documented mainly in the context of starvation, ketone metabolism is not well-understood by most physicians (let alone nutritionists, dietitians, trainers, and athletes) as an approach to improve health and performance. This is primarily due to the emphasis in standard nutrition training placed on dietary carbohydrates as the preferred fuel for physical performance.

## Steve's Keto-Adaptation Experiments in Endurance Athletes

Steve first wandered outside the box three decades ago, performing a pair of studies that established the human capacity to adapt to very low carbohydrate ketogenic diets[6, 14]. One of these experiments was conducted in lean highly trained cyclists ($VO_2$max >65 mL/kg/min) who normally consumed a high carbohydrate diet. The athletes performed an endurance test to exhaustion on their usual diet and then again after being fed a very low carbohydrate diet for 4 weeks. The diet consisted of 1.75 g/kg protein, <10 g carbohydrate, >80% of energy as fat, and was supplemented with minerals including sodium. Riding a stationary cycle at over 900 kcal per hour, the average performance time was almost identical before (147 min) and after (151 min) adapting to the very low carbohydrate diet.

This study demonstrated complete preservation of endurance performance after 4 weeks on a diet that contained virtually no carbohydrate. There was however a dramatic shift in metabolic fuel from a heavy dependence on carbohydrate to nearly complete reliance on fat in the keto-adapted cyclists. The rate of fat use during the exercise test at 64% $VO_2$max was approximately 90 grams per hour (1.5 grams per minute). This is over 3 times the average peak fat oxidation recorded by Venables et al[9] in 300 people that included highly trained individuals with maximal oxygen uptakes exceeding 80 mL/kg/min. Even if you cherry pick and take the participant with the highest peak fat oxidation (60 g fat/hour) observed by Venables et al[9], that value is still less than the keto-adapted participant from Steve's study with the lowest peak fat oxidation (74 g fat/hour). On average keto-adaptation resulted in peak fat oxidation rates of 90 g fat/hour – 50% greater than the highest recorded value for any participant in Venables' study. A couple of Steve's keto-adapted cyclists had fat oxidation rates approaching 2 grams per minute compared to 1 gram per minute when they previously did the same exercise on their high carbohydrate diet. Thus these highly trained athletes, who already had very high fat oxidation rates, were able to dramatically increase them further – not by changing their training, but by changing their diet.

***Factoid:*** *Metabolic adaptations to increase peak fat oxidation can be increased by training, but there remains a large untapped potential in even the most highly trained athlete that can only be achieved by keto-adaptation.*

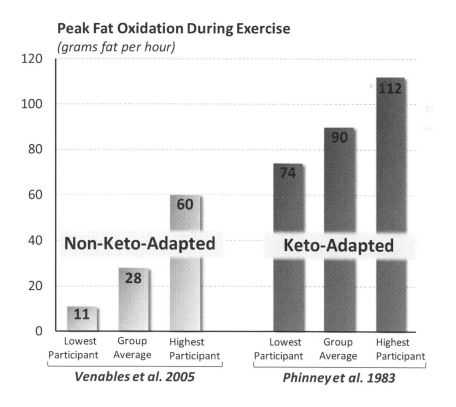

**Peak Fat Oxidation During Exercise**
*(grams fat per hour)*

Despite these intriguing results showing the metabolic plasticity of high level athletes on a very low carbohydrate diet, for a variety of reasons this dietary strategy has languished for three decades. And for the record, it is noteworthy that Steve's findings have not been refuted by additional research over that time period. In fact, subsequent studies in rodents[15] and humans[16] have found similar results.

## Keto-Adaptation De-mystified

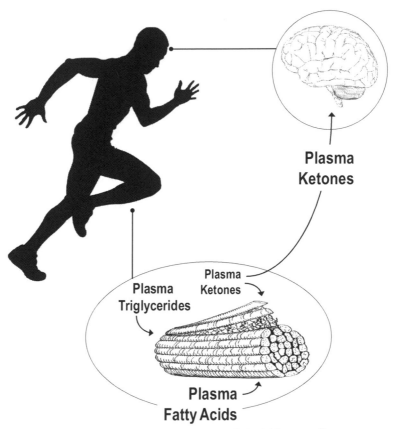

Keto-adaptation results in a powerful shift to reliance on lipid-based fuel sources, especially fatty acids for muscle and ketones for the central nervous system.

At the most basic level keto-adaptation involves an increase in the body's production and utilization of ketones. However, this is a complex and co-ordinated sequence of highly orchestrated events requiring adaptations in the type of fuel used by most cells in the body. Ketone production occurs mainly in the liver in response to a combination of increased delivery of fatty acids and depletion of hepatic glycogen reserves. The ketones produced in the liver are then transported by the circulation to other cells in the body including muscle and brain. In skeletal muscle, the first few days of keto-adaptation result in increased use of both ketones plus fatty acids from a variety of sources (adipose or intra-muscular triglycerides, or from circulating very low density lipoprotein particles). Once the process of keto-adaptation is complete (which takes from a few weeks to a month), muscle both at rest and during exercise comes to rely heavily on fatty acids. This adaptation of the muscle away from ketone use spares hepatic ketone production for use by other tissues, especially the brain.

This is a key point. Practically speaking, the brain can burn only glucose or ketones. On a very low carbohydrate diet, the brain comes to rely on ketones as its primary fuel. Although ketones are preferentially taken up by the brain, because of the large mass of skeletal muscle and the increase in blood flow to active muscles during exercise, this delayed shift of the muscles away from ketones and towards fatty acid use is vital to preserving fuel flow to the brain during exercise in the keto-adapted athlete. In part, the time it takes the body to choreograph these changes in whole body fuel flow explain why keto-adaptation takes a couple of weeks rather than just a few hours or days.

## Jeff's Keto-Adaptation Experiment With Resistance Training

In addition to Steve's keto-adaptation experiments described in the previous section, Jeff has performed studies showing that very low carbohydrate diets can support performance of high intensity resistance exercise, resulting in striking improvements in body composition[17]. Overweight men were randomly assigned to either a low-fat diet group that restricted fat to less than 25% of energy or a very low–carbohydrate ketogenic diet group that reduced carbohydrate to less than 50 grams per day. Half the subjects in each diet group were also randomly assigned to participate in a supervised high intensity resistance training program while the other half of each group remained sedentary.

The training program was 'nonlinear', alternating among heavy, moderate, and light days. Sessions were about 45 minutes in duration performed 3–4 days per week for 12 weeks and included a variety of free weight and machine exercises targeting the entire musculature.

Training loads were determined using repetition maximum (RM) zones (e.g., 1–10 RM) and were progressively increased over the training period. Body composition was assessed using dual energy x-ray absorptiometry. The low carbohydrate diet group lost significantly more body fat, and showed greater decreases in blood insulin levels. Resistance training, independent of diet, resulted in increased lean body mass without compromising fat loss in both diet groups. The most dramatic reduction in percent body fat was in the low-carbohydrate diet plus resistance training group.

**Change in Percent Body Fat**

The combination of a very low carbohydrate diet and resistance training results in the largest decreases in percent body fat.

Thus, the combination of a very low carbohydrate diet and resistance training had a profound effect on body composition by maximizing fat loss while increasing lean body mass.

Individual responses in the low carbohydrate plus resistance training group were dramatic in several cases. One subject lost 20 pounds of fat while gaining 9 pounds of lean body mass. Another one lost 19 pounds of fat while gaining 12 pounds of lean body mass. The greatest fat loss was 30 pounds and this participant gained 9 of pounds lean body mass. In a different study, a 57 year old male (180 pounds, BMI 25 kg/m$^2$) who was training for a triathlon enrolled in a very low carbohydrate study. Following the initial two week period during which his training intensity was reduced, he reported having some of the best training sessions of his life. In just 12 weeks, he lost 23 pounds of fat and gained 6 pounds of lean body mass.

## Summary

During endurance sports, maintaining high carbohydrate availability is challenging, whereas switching to lipid fuels with the selective partitioning of ketones among organs could be revolutionary for athletes. Given the vast differences in the capacities of the 'Fat Tank' versus the 'Glycogen Tank', even a lean person's lipid reserves represent a more plentiful and efficient fuel source. The only thing that stands between you and full access to your body fat stores is a brief period of adaptation to a low carbohydrate diet. Given this background on human metabolism and fuel exchange, we hope it is apparent that a low carbohydrate diet that allows you to optimally access your fat stores and increases mitochondrial fat oxidation is a fully rational approach. In the next chapter we discuss the benefits of keto-adaptation for athletes in greater detail.

# Chapter 4
# KETO-ADAPTATION
*Metabolic Benefits And Sports Implications*

**Snap Shot**

- Keto-adaptation provides a steady and sustained source of fuel for the brain, thereby protecting athletes from hitting the wall.

- Keto-adaptation may improve insulin sensitivity and recovery from exercise.

- Keto-adaptation spares protein from being oxidized thereby preserving lean tissue.

- Keto-adaptation decreases the accumulation of lactate, contributing to better control of pH and respiratory function.

- The benefits of keto-adaptation may be relevant for improving endurance, strength/power, and cognitive performance, as well as speeding recovery.

There are many reasons why people exercise, ranging from recreational, highly competitive, up to professional. Similarly, there are many different reasons you might consider keto-adapting by embracing a low carbohydrate lifestyle. In this chapter we describe some of the potential benefits of keto-adaptation so you have a better appreciation of how following a low carbohydrate lifestyle might impact your unique situation.

## Metabolic Benefits of Keto-Adaptation for Athletes

There are now many studies documenting the metabolic effects of ketosis, although much of this work has been done in the context of short-term starvation, type 2 diabetes, and for neurological disorders like childhood seizures. Less research has been done using ketogenic diets in high level athletes, with the notable exceptions of Steve's and Jeff's original work[6, 17] and that of Tim Noakes[16]. Nevertheless, we now have a good understanding of how well formulated ketogenic diets affect a variety of metabolic parameters in normal-weight and overweight individuals. This work has focused on non-athletes and has consistently shown benefits on a broad spectrum of health markers ranging from cholesterol and lipid values to inflammation, blood pressure, and more. In addition, we now have the practical experience of a growing number of athletes who have adopted a low carbohydrate diet from which to draw inferential conclusions [see Chapter 12]. We present the following discussion to be provocative, fully aware that a complete understanding of how keto-adaptation affects athletic performance remains to be elucidated.

***Brain Fuel***. In order for the body to shift from glucose to fat for fuel, there need to be alterations in inter-organ fuel exchange – the process that partitions lipid fuels to specific sites for oxidation. Although skeletal muscle has the capacity to take up and oxidize ketones, it appears that over time muscles switch to using fatty acids provided from blood and probably muscle triglycerides. This process, a key element of keto-adaptation, allows ketones to achieve levels in the blood that allow them to meet most of the brain's fuel needs. Thus there is a reciprocal relationship between blood ketones and uptake in muscle; such that when blood ketone levels are low, muscle uptake is high, whereas at higher levels, muscle uptake is reduced. The relationship is different in the brain where ketones are rapidly taken up by a combination of passive and facilitated diffusion via monocarboxylic acid transporters in proportion to their concentration in the blood[18, 19].

*Hunch: Since monocarboxylic acid transporters function to take up both ketones and lactate, and they are upregulated in the presence of high ketones, might keto-adaptation result in better handling of lactate (not just through less production but better clearance as well)?*

Thus, when the oxidation of ketones in skeletal muscle is reduced, blood ketones rise. This adaptation facilitates an increase in ketone transport across the blood brain barrier to meet the majority of energy demands of the brain. A low carbohydrate diet that increases ketone levels above 1 millimolar (typical of someone eating less than 50 g/day of total carbs) increases expression of monocarboxylic acid transporters levels eightfold in rat brain cells[18] and also increases brain uptake of ketones by a similar magnitude[19] accounting for over half the brain's fuel use.

One implication of this adaptation is protection from 'hitting the wall', an event primarily associated with inadequate fuel for the brain. This problem (aka 'bonking') occurs in the non-keto-adapted athlete when muscle and liver glycogen reserves are exhausted, leaving muscle and brain to compete for the relatively small amount of glucose that can be made by gluconeogenesis from protein. In addition to improving fuel availability during prolonged exercise, the keto-adapted state may also protect against central fatigue (discussed on page 34). Anecdotally, this sustained supply of fuel to the brain also improves cognition during and after exercise. Besides fuel, ketone bodies have been proposed to have multiple actions in the brain (e.g., providing substrates to help repair damaged neurons, altering membrane potential, etc.). These reported additional metabolic benefits of ketones have prompted a surge in studies of low carbohydrate diets to treat several neurologic disorders (e.g., seizures and Alzheimer's disease).

*Factoid: Many decades ago in a provocative experiment to demonstrate the human brain's ability to function well on ketones, some scientists in Boston keto-adapted 3 obese humans with a month of total starvation. With their BOHB levels around 5 millimolar, they slowly infused insulin into their blood stream over hours until the subjects' blood glucose levels dropped to the point that they should have lapsed into a coma (1.5 millimolar, or less than 30 mg/dl). At that point, their BOHB levels were slightly reduced to 4 millimolar, and not only did they stay awake, these subjects had none of the typical symptoms of hypoglycemia[20].*

***Insulin Sensitivity.*** Exercise sharply increases the rate of production of oxygen free radicals (aka, reactive oxygen species, or ROS). Primary targets of ROS are highly unsaturated fatty acids (HUFA) in cell membranes. Although HUFA are highly susceptible to free radical destruction, we are just beginning to make the connection that exercise-induced increases in ROS could decrease membrane HUFA content. An ROS-mediated destruction of HUFA in membranes would be expected to have an overall deleterious effect on recovery from exercise by impacting metabolic, inflammatory, immune, coagulation and fibrinolytic processes.

This is not purely theoretical. Multiple studies have demonstrated that a low muscle phospholipid HUFA content is related to the level of insulin resistance[21, 22], and thus an important effect of protecting HUFA from ROS-mediated peroxidation is better insulin sensitivity. In untrained subjects, our research shows both improved insulin sensitivity and better membrane HUFA preservation with a low carb diet compared to a high carb diet[23], and we are in the process of examining this effect during high volume exercise as well.

***Hunch:*** *Keto-adaptation may help preserve membrane HUFA, leading to better insulin sensitivity and recovery from exercise.*

***Protein-Sparing.*** In contrast to popular opinion that low carbohydrate diets cause muscle loss and weakness, the objective evidence leads us to the opposite conclusion. This is an important topic that has not received a lot of recent attention by researchers, but the preponderance of evidence clearly indicates that a well formulated ketogenic diet spares the body's protein from oxidation. Infusion of BOHB into healthy adults has been shown to reduce nitrogen excretion during prolonged starvation. This infusion of BOHB is also associated with better maintenance and even increases in circulating branched-chain amino acids (BCAA: leucine, isoleucine, and valine)[24]. The BCAA are classed as 'essential amino acids', which means that they cannot be made from scratch by the body. Thus maintaining adequate levels in the blood is critical for the body's ability to synthesize protein to build or repair organs like muscle or red blood cells.

In Steve's keto-adaptation experiments in cyclists[6], circulating BCAA rose significantly during the ketogenic diet compared to their levels during the baseline high carbohydrate diet. This occurred despite the fact that both diets contained the same amounts of protein. BCAA oxidation typically increases in proportion to energy demands. In keto-adapted athletes, however, there appears to be less need for muscle to use BCAA as fuel, perhaps because the BCAA and ketones have similar 'carbon skeletons' and thus the ketones are burned in place of the BCAA. This was effectively demonstrated by Steve's follow-up study showing that the higher blood leucine levels were a result of markedly decreased leucine oxidation. This finding is consistent with prior work in diaphragm muscle showing that BOHB inhibits the oxidation of leucine[25].

Blood leucine, which increases on a ketogenic diet, is known to be a potent regulator of muscle protein synthesis. Insulin, which decreases on a ketogenic diet, has a permissive role in promoting protein synthesis. Unaware of this counterbalancing effect from increased leucine levels, critics of low carbohydrate diets assumed that reduced insulin levels would cause muscle loss. However the net effect of nutritional ketosis from a well-formulated low carbohydrate diet is at least maintenance of lean body mass despite a much lower insulin level.

In support of a positive effect on retention of skeletal muscle during nutritional ketosis, Young et al[26] compared 3 isocaloric (1,800 kcal/day), isoprotein (115 g) diets differing in carbohydrate content (30, 60, and 104 g) consumed for 9 weeks in obese men. The diet with the lowest amount of carbohydrate (30 g/day) was associated with increased ketones, greater fat loss, and greater preservation of lean tissue compared to the diets with more carbohydrate. Thus, in the keto-adapted state, the body improves its efficiency of protein utilization. The greater economy of protein allows for less to be consumed while still maintaining positive nitrogen balance. This in turn allows for greater production of ketones since consuming too much protein has anti-ketogenic effects.

***Central Fatigue.*** Some ultra-marathon athletes are now training and competing on low carbohydrate regimens, and one advantage they cite is less central fatigue (i.e., fatigue from altered brain function, resulting in confusion and depression) late in their events (See Chapter 12). It is feasible that this is due to better preservation of BCAA across prolonged exercise, resulting in less brain aromatic amino acid uptake. The central fatigue theory posits that a relative increase in the blood level of tryptophan accelerates transport of this amino acid across the blood brain barrier. Tryptophan is used by the brain to make 5-hydroxytryptamine (aka serotonin) , a neurotransmitter that depresses neuronal activity leading to fatigue. Tryptophan competes for transport into the brain with other neutral amino acids (particularly BCAA), and therefore maintaining higher blood levels of leucine will cause less tryptophan uptake and therefore less serotonin production by the brain[27].

***Lactate Metabolism.*** An increased reliance on fat and a corresponding decrease in glycolysis during exercise is associated with less accumulation of lactate (a surrogate for hydrogen ion accumulation). As cellular lactate and hydrogen ion levels increase at higher intensities of exercise, there are several events that cause force production and work capacity to decrease. A key contributor in this process is the acidity (i.e., decreasing pH) associated with hydrogen ion buildup. Along with maximal oxygen consumption, lactate threshold (the exercise intensity where blood lactate begins to accumulate) is a major determinant of endurance performance. With the enhanced ability to oxidize lipid associated with keto-adaptation, there is less lactate production at any one workload, and thus an elevation in the threshold exercise intensity associated with increased acidity.

***Ventilatory Drive.*** There are two primary drivers of your respiration. The first is the blood oxygen level – you breathe harder if the brain perceives a low oxygen content in the blood. The second driver is carbon dioxide, which drops the blood pH (makes it more acid) when $CO_2$ accumulates, and this reduced blood pH increases respiration. This is also why having lactic acid build up in the blood during intense anaerobic exercise causes such intense hyper-ventilation, because its buildup also contributes to a drop in blood pH.

Once you are adapted to a low carb diet, two things influencing your respiratory drive change. First, your respiratory quotient (RQ) at most workloads is lower, which means you make less $CO_2$ per calorie burned, so there's less of a pH drop and less respiratory drive. Ditto that for lactate as well – at most workloads all the way to your max output, lactate levels are also lower. Obviously you still need to breathe hard enough to get the oxygen you need into your blood to perform the work, but under most circumstances you are protected from that intense sense of 'air hunger' that comes from having dropped your blood pH into the basement.

**Factoid:** *RQ is the ratio of $CO_2$ expired to $O_2$ consumed. Burning exclusively carbs results in equal amounts of $CO_2$ expired to $O_2$ consumed, and thus an RQ = 1.0. Burning exclusively fat results in an RQ of 0.7(i.e., only 70% as much $CO_2$ expired as when burning glucose). In a keto-adapted athlete, most endurance exercise is done at RQ values less than 0.75.*

One of the many myths about ketogenic diets is that they cause the body to go into a state of acidosis. This stems from the unfortunate fact that many doctors and lay people alike confuse nutritional ketosis (blood ketones at 1-3 millimolar) with keto-acidosis (blood ketones greater than 20 millimolar). In nutritional ketosis, blood pH at rest stays normal, plus sharp drops in pH due to $CO_2$ and lactate buildup during exercise are restrained. By contrast, in keto-acidosis, blood pH is driven abnormally low by the 10-fold greater buildup of ketones. Suggesting these two states are similar is like equating a gentle rain with a flood because they both involve water.

One way we doctors traditionally make the diagnosis of diabetic keto-acidosis in the emergency room is simply observing a patient lying at rest on a gurney but puffing like someone who just finished a 100-meter dash. This hyperventilation at rest is driven by their very high blood ketone levels – something that never happens as a result of nutritional ketosis.

And there you have the paradox of nutritional ketosis – blood pH and respiration are actually better controlled when your body has adapted to ketone-based energy flow, even though ketones are technically acid compounds.

## Sports Implications

The direct metabolic benefits of keto-adaptation translate into two general effects relevant to most athletes.

1.  Improved body composition (power-to-weight ratio)
2.  Improved prolonged endurance performance resulting from better sustained fuel delivery

*Improved Body Composition.* Being overweight or obese usually means carrying excess adipose tissue. If you want to lose 'weight', what you really want to do is lose body fat. There are many good reasons for losing body fat for general health and well-being, even if you don't consider yourself overweight or metabolically sick.

- Decreasing adipose tissue may help you maintain a specific body weight as a requirement of your sport (e.g., wrestling, boxing, powerlifting, Olympic lifting, judo, mixed martial arts, etc.) or for sports where physical appearance is a component of success (e.g., bodybuilding, gymnastics, dancing, fitness model competitions, figure skating, platform diving, etc.).

- Decreasing body fat while maintaining or even building muscle mass may translate into a greater quickness, agility, and performance. From a functional perspective, body fat is not involved in force production and therefore decreasing body fat does not adversely affect strength or power production. In fact a loss in body fat, and therefore body weight, improves your power to weight ratio, a key determinant of both acceleration and endurance performance. Think about 2 cyclists climbing a hill who have the same pedaling power, but one weighs 200 lbs and the other 175 lbs. Who gets to the top first? Clearly the lighter athlete since s/he has less total weight and therefore less total work to perform. A higher power to weight ratio also translates into greater speed and quickness which is relevant for athletes who participate in sports demanding short high-intensity and explosive bursts.

- If ridding yourself of even a little body fat improves your self-perception (i.e., you feel better about your body), your head is in a better place going into your game.

If losing body fat is a goal, you might have tried a calorically-restricted, low-fat, high-carbohydrate diet only to find yourself feeling constantly hungry, drained, and unable to complete your workouts. Such low-fat weight loss diets often provide just enough carbohydrate to prevent keto-adaptation but not enough to fuel exercise. The result compromises workout volume/intensity, recovery ability, and training adaptations. A better approach is to give your muscle and brain cells optimized access to your fat stores by becoming keto-adapted. This strategy provides adequate energy to fuel exercise without ever putting your fat cells into storage mode. Thus a well formulated low carbohydrate diet is ideal for targeting fat loss without compromising training intensity and adaptations.

**Factoid:** *Body fat (aka adipose tissue) consists of cells that are roughly 15% lean tissue (i.e., cellular 'machinery' like mitochondria and the nucleus) and 85% fat in one big central droplet.*

In the past, it was assumed that fat cells lived 'forever', but now we know that they die off intermittently and are replaced by new fat cells as needed. Thus losing body fat means reducing not just the fat droplet size, but also the amount of the associated 'machinery'. This means that for each 10 pounds of body fat you lose, about 8.5 pounds is actual 'fat', while 1.5 pounds is considered lean tissue based on various tests like density (underwater weighing, the BodPod), electrical impedance, or DXA. Therefore, if you lose 10 pounds on a well-formulated low carb diet and before and after DXA tests indicate that you have the same lean body mass, this means that you have actually gained 1.5 pounds of lean tissue somewhere else than in your fat cells.

***Improved Prolonged Endurance Performance and Cognition.*** In the non-keto-adapted athlete, a key element contributing to deteriorating performance (both physical and mental) during prolonged exercise is reduced carbohydrate availability. This results in a crisis in fuel flow because of the body's inability to promptly adapt to utilizing body fat stores as an alternative fuel source, particularly for the brain. Since humans have a limited capacity to store carbohydrate, this requires that endurance athletes frequently consume carbohydrates to support their high rates of carbohydrate oxidation during prolonged exercise. This poses obvious logistical problems, both in having timely access to carbohydrate foods/supplements and in maintaining adequate digestive function to allow their absorption without undue gastro-intestinal side effects. For these reasons, optimizing body fat oxidation represents a more sustainable and efficient source of fuel for better physical and mental performance and enhanced recovery. Armed with a heightened ability to access and utilize a much larger (and thus more sustainable) fuel source, the most obvious performance advantage would be during workouts or competitions that last more than 2 hours (i.e., athletes training for marathons, triathlons, or any ultra-endurance events).

In addition to direct metabolic effects during a workout or competition, proper restriction of dietary carbohydrate can lead to several positive outcomes relevant to recovery for athletes. This is discussed in Chapter 5.

## Side Bar: The Uncomfortable Truth About Endurance Exercise, Resting Energy Expenditure, and Weight Loss

Here is an excellent question we've received on occasion from careful readers of our book: 'The Art and Science of Low Carbohydrate Living' (aka LCL).

Our answer, however, is about as uncomfortable as an answer can get. Perhaps you are thinking we are about to say "we don't know". Sorry, because as scientists we love that kind of answer. "I DON'T KNOW" is like a billboard flashing the message "DO RESEARCH HERE!"

No, we are uncomfortable with our answer because we know that you probably won't like it, and that hell will have to freeze over before many people (including many experts in the field) will accept it. But that said, with the excuse that a few of you asked for it, here goes.

There are 4 well-controlled, inpatient, metabolic ward studies (the gold standard for human research) published from 1982 thru 1997 that showed statistically significant reductions in resting metabolic rate when overweight subjects performed 300-600 Calories per day of endurance exercise for weeks at a time[28-31]. There are no equally rigorous human studies showing the opposite. There are animal (rat) studies that show the opposite, and there are human studies done under less controlled conditions that show the opposite. However there are also similarly less rigorous studies that agree with the above four gold-standard studies. When the quality/rigor of the studies is taken into account, the weight of the evidence supports two main conclusions:

1.  Humans vary one-from-another in how their metabolism responds to endurance exercise, and much of this inter-individual variation is inherited (genetic). Given this wide individual variance, studies involving small numbers of subjects could get differing results based on random chance.

2.  Although genetically lean people as a group may respond differently, when overweight humans do more than one hour of endurance exercise daily, resting metabolism on average declines between 5 and 15%.

The fascinating question is, if our interpretation of this published literature turns out to be correct, then how come most doctors, dietitians, and sports scientists think the opposite? Part of the answer is that there is a lot of simple logic suggesting that exercise speeds resting metabolism. First, exercise builds muscle, and muscle burns energy even at rest. Second, there are a lot of skinny athletes out there who think they are skinny because they train hard (as opposed to being able to train hard because they are skinny). Third, it is a common observation that heavy people tend not to exercise much, so it is easy to blame their weight problem on a lack of exercise. And finally, everyone loves a '2-for-the-price-of-one' sale. It's just way too tempting to think that you could burn 600 Calories during a 1-hour run and then, as a result, burn another 600 Calories over the course of the next day?

The other factor contributing to the experts' non-acceptance of our interpretation of the published data is something we have named "The Warren and Marshall Syndrome" ([1]pages 177-8). Back in the 1980s Drs. Warren and Marshall discovered that a bacterium causes stomach ulcers – not acid like everybody thought. For more than a decade, their brilliant research was ignored or dismissed by the 'medical experts'. In the meantime, people suffered needlessly, had major surgery, and even died from bleeding ulcers that could have been cured by a few weeks of inexpensive antibiotics. Finally, in the mid-1990s the medical profession 'flipped' and suddenly curing ulcers with antibiotics became the hot new thing (and later on Drs. Warren and Marshall got their justly deserved Nobel Prize).

So why did it take so long? One reason might be that people (especially those who consider themselves experts) don't like to change their minds. And then too, there were huge economic forces against this change – billions of dollars of antacid medications were being sold, and thousands of surgeons were kept busy cutting out the ulcers. Nobody (well, accept the patients with ulcers) wanted to see this massive revenue stream suddenly dry up.

Fast-forward to the issue at hand. What would happen if the public was told that, for many of us, exercise doesn't speed your metabolism and that it doesn't do that much to speed weight loss? Yes, some people would still run marathons and go to gyms to work out. But those would be the folks who actually enjoy doing vigorous exercise. The heavy people who were shamed into joining the gym or pounding the pavement in $100 shoes hoping to melt off their excess pounds, however, would more likely (from the marketing perspective) just melt away.

We are not saying that exercise isn't good for people. Both of us are personally committed to leading vigorous lives, and encouraging others to consider doing the same. What we object to, however, is misinforming the public as to what and how much benefit they can expect from exercise, particularly as it pertains to weight loss. From our perspective, telling heavy people to exercise because it speeds resting metabolism (and thus markedly increaseing one's rate of weight loss) is about as credible as selling them the Brooklyn Bridge.

# Chapter 5

# EXERCISE RECOVERY

*Returning Rapidly To Full Function*

## Snap Shot

- Avoiding wide excursions in blood sugar and in-sulin by burning predominately fatty acids and ke-tones can lessen the 'stress' response to exercise.

- Keto-adaptation results in less generation of reactive oxygen species (ROS) and therefore better preserva-tion of highly unsaturated fatty acids (HUFA) in cell membranes.

- Less metabolic stress, improved fuel flow, and healthier membranes translate into faster recovery from exercise and less exercise-induced inflamma-tion, immunosupression, gastro-intestinal distress, insulin resistance, muscle damage, and soreness.

- Maintaining adequate membrane HUFA status can be further supported by ensuring adequate intake (via your diet or supplements) of omega-3 HUFA and antioxidant/anti-inflammatory compounds like the 'gamma form' of vitamin E.

The body's response to exercise is fascinating and complex. Researchers, including ourselves, have studied recovery from exercise by measuring various metabolites, hormones, membrane components, inflammatory signals, immune cells, and markers of oxidative stress and muscle damage. What do we know about recovery? The answer is a lot. What do we *not* know about recovery? The answer is a lot more. We won't try to review the body of work done on recovery, but instead provide you an innovative perspective on the potential benefits of keto-adaptation on important recovery processes.

## Ketogenic Diets and Oxidative Stress

A provocative way to think about ketones is that they are a clean-burning fuel, in that their production and oxidation appears to result in less generation of reactive oxygen species (ROS) compared to other metabolic substrates like glucose and glycogen. ROS (aka oxygen free radicals) are highly reactive molecules produced by mitochondria that damage tissue proteins and membrane polyunsaturated fats. Previous work has shown that BOHB levels in the blood within the range of nutritional ketosis (1-3 millimolar) decreases mitochondrial ROS production[32] and increase antioxidant defenses[33].

ROS are tightly linked to inflammation and aging. We have published data demonstrating that a well-formulated low carbohydrate diet reduces levels of systemic inflammation[23]. In contrast, exercise increases ROS production[34], and we have preliminary evidence that prolonged intense exercise (even in highly trained athletes) can overwhelm systemic antioxidant defenses and degrade membrane essential fatty acid content. This in turn could explain both impaired immune function and loss of gastrointestinal integrity commonly observed after prolonged exercise. Thus it is likely that another benefit of a well formulated low carbohydrate diet is that by reducing oxidative stress and inflammation, gut and immune functions are better maintained. If this is bourne out by research we have in progress, it can explain many of the benefits in recovery reported by pioneering athletes who have adopted a low carbohydrate lifestyle.

In support of this hypothesis, Steve and our colleague Dr. Doug Bibus obtained data from racing sled dogs (remember those Super Fat-Burning Athletes at the end of Chapter 2). In 2005, Steve and Doug analyzed blood and cheek swabs from a small number of dogs from three teams before and after 1000 miles of competition. It was our hypothesis that the cumulative oxidative stress in these dogs would degrade membrane phospholipid essential fatty acids (MP-EFA), and that this effect over 10 days would be better observed in cheek cells (fast cell turnover) compared to red blood cells (slow cell turnover). It turns out there were considerable differences in the observed changes in membranes between racing teams (suggesting major diet effects), but we did not know the diet compositions for these teams. As anticipated, there was little change in red blood cell MP-EFA, however all teams showed numerical reductions in one or more classes of cheek cell MP-EFA. In one team, these reductions in both omega-3 and omega-6 MP-EFA classes were greater than 50%. A second team demonstrated intermediate changes, and one team had little or no changes. Our interim conclusions are that gut membranes (i.e., cheek cells) are subject to dramatic alterations due to oxidative stress from prolonged exercise, and that diet is potentially a potent moderator of this effect.

## Insulin Sensitivity

It is well known that exercise improves the insulin sensitivity of muscle cells, and as a group, highly trained endurance athletes tend to be uniformly very insulin sensitive. A decade ago, however, a Finnish research group studied insulin sensitivity and muscle glycogen recovery in a group of runners after completing a marathon[35]. To their surprise, they discovered these runners to be more insulin resistant in the first few days after the marathon than they were before the race, and this occurred despite their muscles still being mostly empty of glycogen. This presents a very interesting paradox – just when we'd expect them to be most insulin sensitive and rapidly rebuilding glycogen reserves, the post-marathon body appears to have run into a temporary metabolic roadblock.

This observation, called the 'post-marathon paradox', has been confirmed by other scientists[36], but perhaps because it remains unexplained, it does not get much attention these days. This is unfortunate, because understanding why this happens and how to counteract it would be very important to optimizing recovery in athletes after high volume training or competition. It is in this context that our preliminary observations of membrane HUFA damage in Iditarod sled dogs may represent a breakthrough in explaining the post-marathon paradox.

As noted in Chapter 4, membrane HUFA are tightly linked with insulin sensitivity, so even a transient reduction in these essential fatty acids in muscle membranes after intense exercise could impair insulin sensitivity and thus limit the rate of recovery. And if, as we suspect, the keto-adapted runner is better protected against this tissue damage, we will have an explanation for the reports of runners claiming more rapid recovery when they train and compete on a low carb regimen (see Chapter 12).

## ROS versus HUFA

***Factoid:*** *Ultra-endurance athletes utilize a surprising amount of oxygen in a short time period. Assuming that trail-running consumes 100-125 Calories per mile, a 100-mile event causes the body to utilize 7 pounds (over 3 kg) of oxygen.*

A small fraction (1-3%) of the oxygen used by mitochondria generates ROS. Most of these ROS should be captured and quenched by anti-oxidant defenses such as superoxide dismutase (SOD), glutathione, and tocopherols (vitamin E). All of these require either replacement or regeneration, however, which means they can be overwhelmed by some combination of poor diet and/or a high volume of ROS production. Assuming a 2% rate of ROS leakage from mitochondria, a 100 mile trail run would generate 63 grams of ROS that must be either quenched or 'absorbed' by nearby tissue. At 32 grams per mole of the most common form of ROS, this translates to 2 moles of highly destructive compounds capable of 'burning' (think 'sunburn') vulnerable molecules.

Some of the most highly vulnerable nearby molecules are membrane HUFA such as arachidonic acid or DHA. These HUFA have molecular weights in the 300-330 grams per mole range, which means that a mole (32 grams) of ROS can destroy 10-times its weight in HUFA. So here's the problem – a pair of well-trained runners legs might contain 200 grams of membrane HUFA, while the ROS produced in those legs in a 100-mile run has the potential to destroy 600 grams of HUFA. Putting this another way, if only 15% of that ROS escaped the body's anti-oxidant containment, it would still be enough to destroy half of the HUFA in that runner's leg muscles. Based on published human muscle data [21, 22], even a 25% reduction in muscle membrane HUFA would dramatically reduce insulin sensitivity.

## Countermeasures Against HUFA Destruction

Like so many other aspects of nutrition, one needs to deal with a 'forest' of factors rather than a single 'tree'. Thus focusing on a single nutrient such as dietary arachidonate, the zinc and copper needed to make super oxide dismutase (SOD – a key enzyme that quenches ROS), or how much and which type of vitamin E to take may be scientifically correct but physiologically inadequate. To optimally reduce HUFA destruction and then speed recovery from that HUFA damage which does occur, we need to consider all of the following:

- Ketogenic diets repeatedly have demonstrated increased proportions of HUFA in serum phospholipid (PL), which means that you would be starting the event with higher HUFA levels.

- Our research indicates that the higher PL HUFA associated with a ketogenic diet is due to a slower rate of destruction rather than making more of them per se. During prolonged exercise, this would translate to less total HUFA destruction (e.g., 30 grams in 100 miles rather than closer to 60 grams as hypothesized above).

- Consuming enough omega-3 HUFA in the diet or as supplements to maintain optimum tissue levels.

- Maintaining a modest intake of anti-inflammatory tocopherols (gamma and delta) as opposed to supplements of highly enriched alpha-tocopherol.

- Eating enough natural meats, fish, and vegetables to get adequate minerals and trace minerals.

- Avoid taking extra iron (even the amount in a 'standard multivitamin' unless you have been diagnosed as iron deficient by your physician.

**Factoid:** *There are 7 common forms of 'vitamin E'. The one that is most potent as an anti-oxidant (alpha-tocopherol) dominates the supplement market. However gamma-tocopherol is a reasonably good anti-oxidant plus it has potent anti-inflammatory properties[37, 38].*

# Section 2

# IMPLEMENTING YOUR DIET PLAN

# Chapter 6

# CARBOHYDRATE

*Why It Is Unnecessary And How To Restrict It*

## Snap Shot

- Although variable from person to person, to get your blood ketones above 1 millimolar typically requires that you  consume less than 50 grams of carbohydrate per day.

- In the context of a well-formulated ketogenic diet, this level of carbohydrate restriction is safe, sustainable, and satisfying.

- As you become aware of the carbohydrate content of foods, you'll discover that an appealing variety of meals can be consumed even at this low level of carbohydrate intake.

- Whereas consuming fast-digesting carbohydrates after exercise is commonly recommended, this practice is counter-productive in the keto-adapted state.

- Once keto-adapted, depending on your metabolism and goals, you may be able to incorporate slow release sources of carbohydrate such as root vegetables, legumes, or UCAN's SuperStarch™.

## Is a Low Carbohydrate Diet Practical and Sustainable?

Before we discuss the practical details of constructing a well formulated ketogenic diet, we need to address a question that will undoubtedly cross many readers' minds:

> ### *Can athletes actually maintain a diet high in fat and low in carbohydrate for extended periods of time?*

The answer is an emphatic **YES**! But the chances that you can stick with it and experience success depends on both your mindset going in and also the quality of the advice you receive on how to formulate your diet. You may have already noted our use of the term 'well-formulated low carbohydrate diet'. There are many versions of low carbohydrate diets promoted in books for lay readers. In our opinion, some are pretty good while others leave us scratching our heads. One simple test is if the book tells you to restrict carbs but doesn't tell you what to eat in their place, that diet is unsustainable. Why? Especially for a lean athlete who doesn't have much body fat to lose, you've got to get your fuel from somewhere. The amount you don't get from carbs has to come from some other practical energy source. To avoid this pitfall, these next three chapters will guide you to the right mix of fuels to consume if you are restricting carbs.

We feel strongly that if you are going down the low carb path, there are certain aspects of the diet that you need to understand to ensure safety, sustainability, and success. That's why we encourage you to read our recent full-length book 'The Art and Science of Low Carbohydrate Living'[1] which provides more background on these topics. In the interest of space, we will highlight the salient features of a well-formulated low-carbohydrate diet in the next several chapters, and then let you flesh out the background as your curiosity dictates.

First a brief word on mindset. We sincerely hope and predict that many athletes who adopt the principles of this book will make permanent changes in their dietary habits and feel empowered as a result. Not everyone who reads this book will have a life-changing experience, but some might and that may include you. Between us we have decades of clinical and personal experience with low carbohydrate diets. This experience extends far beyond the transient "fad use" of carbohydrate restriction for weight loss. Both of us personally, and many of our patients as well, have spent many years in uninterrupted nutritional ketosis. This experience leads us to the firm conclusion that with a modicum of support and counseling, human subjects, patients, and athletes alike can be guided through keto-adaptation to a reasonably simple and satisfying weight maintaining low carbohydrate diet. Although not commonly appreciated or practiced, our research and practical experience with low carbohydrate diets has revealed important insights into the appropriate quantity and quality of fats, minerals, and micronutrients needed to ensure a palatable and sustainable low carbohydrate life-style. So what about mindset? If you don't believe that a low carb lifestyle is safe or sustainable, it probably won't be. However we hope that that amount and quality of the information we provide you empowers you with the confidence you need to allow this dietary strategy to work for you.

*Factoid: Within the class of nutrients called 'carbohydrates', there is no molecule that is essential for human health or well-being. This does not mean that blood sugar is completely unimportant, but rather that blood sugar can be well-maintained via metabolic processes such as gluconeogenesis without dietary carbohydrates in the keto-adapted human.*

## Cutting Carbs

If this is your first time launching into a low carbohydrate/high-fat diet, you are in for a bit of an adjustment. On its surface, cutting out most dietary carbs may sound simple, but that ignores our strong cultural ties to (and perhaps biochemical dependence on) carbohydrates. You have the best chance of success if you educate yourself as much as possible on the carbohydrate and fat contents of the foods you currently eat. It also helps to develop a shopping list to make sure you have a variety of alternative low-carbohydrate foods on hand. Given this preparation and a modest amount of effort, over time you will better understand how to incorporate your favorite ingredients, recipes and dishes into your new lifestyle. Here we provide a broad overview of the key principles of the diet. For additional details, including specific strategies and recipes for increasing the right types of fat, we highly recommend reading Chapter 17 (The Joy of Cooking and Eating Fat) from "The Art and Science of Low Carbohydrate Living"[1].

## How Low to Go

Inducing a state of nutritional ketosis and maintaining it long enough to complete keto-adaptation requires a conscientious effort to restrict carbohydrates for two or more weeks. The level of carbohydrate restriction required to optimize fat burning and fat loss varies from person to person, but the most consistent effects will be achieved at levels of carbohydrate below 50 grams per day. If this sounds frightening to you, that's understandable because you may be accustomed to consuming up to 10 times that amount. Don't despair, however – this is not as restrictive as you may think. Even 50 grams per day of carbohydrate opens the door to eating copious amounts of low-carbohydrate/high-fat, highly satiating and satisfying foods.

In addition to reducing your dietary carbs, an important factor for getting into nutritional ketosis is to not over-consume protein. This is explained in detail in the next chapter, but suffice it to say that cutting your carbs means eating more fat rather than two steaks when you give up that side of a baked potato or rice pilaf. Once you are keto-adapted, you will likely experience a surprising appreciation for fat and heightened pleasure associated with eating fat-containing foods. Many athletes who have gone through this process note that it is empowering not having to count calories while decreasing body fat and enjoying an uninterrupted flow of energy.

## How Fast to Cut Back?

This is a great question, but the answer is not as clearly spelled out by objective research as we would like. Some very credible people advocate easing into carbohydrate restriction slowly by cutting back by one food category at a time (e.g., first sugars and juices, then refined carbs, then starchy vegetables, etc). Others take the 'Nike approach' – as in "just do it". To date, no one has done a study with a large group of subjects to see which strategy yields a higher proportion making an effective transition into nutritional ketosis.

What we do know is that it takes a couple of weeks to keto-adapt, and you don't accomplish much towards that goal until you are making substantial amounts of ketones (i.e., eating less than 50 grams of carbs for most people). The other concern with easing into a low carb diet is that once you are eating less than the 150 grams of carb needed to feed your brain with glucose, but still more than the 50 gram threshold below which ketosis is dependably operating, your brain's fuel supply becomes pretty tenuous. If there's not enough glucose to meet the brain's 600 Calorie daily energy habit, and blood ketones remain below the 0.5 millimolar threshold where they can begin to pitch in, your body's only two options are:

    a)   burn up protein (for gluconeogenesis to fill the gap) or
    b)   binge on carbs.

In our clinical experience, the 'Nike approach' is better. Particularly if you use broth/bouillon to get enough sodium and eat plenty of low carb vegetables to get enough potassium, your adaptation period will be short and relatively symptom-free. That does not mean that this transition will be easy, but perhaps easier that trying to slowly slide your metabolism between two distinctly different fueling strategies. The best analogy might be that when running a gauntlet, it's better to pick your antagonists armed with whips than those armed with hatchets.

## Getting Below 50

Where does this daily allotment of (give or take) 50 grams of carbohydrate come from? Well, for starters, when it comes to cereals, breads, pasta, potatoes, pastry, candy, juices, or other carb-dense foods we'll say it once…just don't go there. Because all of these are like the ***nuclear option*** in suppressing ketones, we've started calling them '***carbage***'. However, here's where you can go. Based on food preferences, availability, and individual tolerance, the exact breakdown will vary from person to person and day to day. But generally, your daily carbohydrate count should total something like this:

- 5-10 grams from protein-based food
- 10-15 grams from vegetables
- 5-10 grams from nuts/seeds
- 5-10 grams from fruits
- 5-10 grams from miscellaneous sources

## Protein-Based Foods (5-10 grams carbs/day)

Meats and cheeses have virtually no carbohydrate with the exception of small amounts in glycogen and lactose, respectively. Therefore most unprocessed meats, fish, and poultry are acceptable as long as you use common sense and avoid versions that contain added carbohydrates (e.g., breaded or heavily seasoned meats with added sugars, starch fillers, or sweet sauces). Read labels and check for hidden carbohydrates that often lurk in meat loaf, hot dogs, sausage, jerky, or cold cuts. Avoid wherever possible highly processed proteins such as hot dogs and 'American cheese'. Why? Processing deletes much of the protein, not to mention associated beneficial nutrients like potassium and magnesium that your muscles need to work properly. Look, for example, at this comparison of what you get from 180 Calories of hot dogs versus the same amount of steak.

| Food | Protein (grams) | Calories | Potassium (mg) | Magnesium (mg) |
|---|---|---|---|---|
| Hot Dog (2 oz) | 7 | 180 | 94 | 2 |
| Round Steak (3 oz) | 26 | 180 | 368 | 26 |

Meats can be marinated with a variety of condiments including olive oil, lemon juice, soy sauce, 'dry' wine, vinegar, garlic and various spices. Do not purposely seek out lean cuts and do not worry about trimming visible fat as this will likely contribute to over-consumption of protein relative to fat. You actually need the fat to fuel your body, and the type found in meats is very suitable, plus it contributes to flavor and satiety. Whole eggs contain about half a gram of carbohydrate each and can be used frequently. You can fry, poach, scramble, or boil eggs or make an omelet.

Select hard cheeses or cream cheese with less than 1 gram of carbohydrate per ounce. Cream (half & half, light or heavy whipping cream) can be used in place of milk for coffee, protein shakes, smoothies, etc. Search for a plain Greek yogurt or unsweetened live culture plain yogurt made from whole milk containing 10-16 grams of carbohydrate per cup. Add your own vanilla or squeeze the juice from a lemon for flavor. Try stirring in butter or cream cheese to add additional texture and fat, and if you want a touch of sweetness add xylitol or Splenda. Yogurt is also an excellent base for salad dressings.

Although the total carbohydrates in yogurt may seem on the high side, in naturally fermented yogurt (the stuff that doesn't contain gelatin), much of this 'carbohydrate' was lactose that has since been converted to lactic acid. This is what makes it taste sour and causes the protein to curdle (i.e., how yogurt changes from a liquid milk to a solid). Eating lactate as opposed to lactose does not raise insulin or interfere with ketosis. Thus a half cup of naturally fermented yogurt counts as about 5 grams of carbs. Avoid fat-free, low-fat, or reduced-fat cheeses and yogurts. Cottage and ricotta (non-fermented) cheeses should be used sparingly.

## Vegetables (10-15 grams carbs/day)

These should appear on your plate at every meal. You can enjoy many different types of vegetables but avoid the starchy ones like potatoes, yams, sweet potatoes, corn, carrots, beets, dried beans and peas. A short list of recommended vegetables that can be frequently consumed includes:

Asparagus
Broccoli (head and raab varieties)
Celery
Cucumber
Cauliflower
Chard
Collards
Eggplant
Endive
Green beans
Kale
Mushrooms
Mustard green
Lettuce (all varieties)
Onions
Pea pods (snow and snap varieties)
Peppers
Radish
Spinach
Summer squash (zucchini and crookneck)

## Nuts and Seeds (5-10 grams carbs/day)

Most nuts, nut butters, and seeds contain about 4-8 grams of carbohydrate per ounce so limit yourself to 2 ounces per day. Nuts can be dry roasted, oil roasted, raw, blanched, chopped, slivered, shelled, salted or unsalted. Avoid honey roasted, barbecued, candy coated, or other varieties with added carbohydrate. Natural peanut butters without added sugars are preferred.

## Fruits (5-10 grams carbs/day)

Berries (e.g., rasp-, straw-, blue-, etc), tomatoes, olives and avocados are relatively low in carbohydrate and packed with nutrients. A daily total of up to 100 grams (3.5 oz) of these berry fruits can be consumed. These are fruits that contain less than 10% by weight total carbs, so 3.5 oz (about half a cup, or 100 grams) provides less than 10 grams. Most other fruits are too high in carbohydrates (despite whatever fiber they contain), and fruit juices (other than tomato juice and V8) are concentrated forms of carbohydrates and should be avoided.

## A Note on Sweeteners

There are lots of opinions vis-a-vis sweeteners for health and performance. We will leave that important debate for another venue. In the context of a low carbohydrate diet, however, do not use 'traditional' sugars like sucrose (table sugar), glucose, fructose, or their aliases (e.g., honey, maple syrup, corn syrup).

As you are no doubt aware, there are a growing number of sugar substitutes that have fewer calories than sucrose that might be appropriate on a low carbohydrate diet. Saccharin (sold as Sweet'N Low in pink packets), aspartame (sold as Equal and NutraSweet in blue packets), and sucralose (sold as Splenda in yellow packets) are many times sweeter than sugar. They can be used in small amounts, and contain virtually zero Calories. Although not as widely distributed in the United States, Stevia (sold as

PureVia, Reb-A, Rebiana, SweetLeaf, and Truvia) is gaining in popularity as a natural no calorie sugar substitute.

Another group of sugars worth discussing are the sugar alcohols which appear in a variety of low carbohydrate products. As shown in the table below, sugar alcohols contain fewer calories than sucrose. Because they are partially absorbed, however, they do provide some energy. The different sugar alcohols vary in calorie content, sweetness, absorption, and perhaps most import their impact on blood glucose and insulin. Maltitol, a common sugar alcohol used in many low carbohydrate products, consistently increases blood glucose and insulin because it has an average glycemic index of 36. Use low carbohydrate products with maltitol sparingly, or better yet stay away from them all together.

Other sugar alcohols have virtually no impact on blood glucose and insulin. Since a portion of most ingested sugar alcohols pass through the gastrointestinal tract unabsorbed, there is the potential for fermentation by bacteria and subsequent bloating, abdominal pain, flatulence, or diarrhea. Thus, as a rule we don't advocate consuming a lot use sugar alcohols. But if you do, we prefer xylitol.

Xylitol is a five carbon sugar alcohol with approximately the same sweetness as sugar and just over half the calories. It has virtually no impact on blood glucose and insulin, and unlike other sugar alcohols, it has nutritive value. Studies show xylitol promotes dental and gut health, has anti-bacterial/anti-microbial effects, and in one recent study animals fed xylitol showed decreased visceral fat mass[39].

| Sugar Alcohol | Kcal/g | Sweetness | Glycemic Index | Absorption (g/100 g) | Fermentation (g/100 g) | Urinary Excretion (g/100 g) |
|---|---|---|---|---|---|---|
| Sucrose | 4.0 | 100% | 60 | 100 | | 0 |
| Erythritol | 0.2 | 70% | 0 | 90 | 10 | 90 |
| Xylitol | 2.5 | 100% | 13 | 50 | 50 | <2 |
| Maltitol | 2.7 | 75% | 36 | 40 | 60 | <2 |
| Isomalt | 2.1 | 55% | 9 | 10 | 90 | <2 |
| Sorbitol | 2.5 | 60% | 9 | 25 | 75 | <2 |
| Lacitol | 2.0 | 35% | 6 | 2 | 98 | <2 |
| Mannitol | 1.5 | 60% | 0 | 25 | 75 | 25 |

## Post-Exercise Carbohydrates

After a hard workout or competition, it is commonly believed that consumption of quickly absorbed, insulin-stimulating carbohydrates are needed to promote glycogen synthesis. The argument that you need a high carbohydrate intake and high insulin levels to replete glycogen reserves is a moot point if you are keto-adapted, since your use of glycogen during exercise will be dramatically reduced. This would be like worrying about putting regular gasoline in your tank when your vehicle has a diesel engine. Furthermore, we are beginning to learn that there are other more subtle downsides associated with consuming insulin-stimulating carbohydrates after exercise.

*Factoid: Consuming even small amounts of carbohydrate after exercise rapidly decreases the release of fatty acids from fat stores and oxidation of fat in the muscle[40], thereby interfering with keto-adaption, plus also diminishing the beneficial effects of exercise on insulin sensitivity and other cardio-metabolic risk markers[41, 42].*

For some athletes, a carbohydrate-induced insulin surge results in a rebound low blood sugar and subsequent stress response characterized by increased counter-regulatory hormones (e.g., epinephrine and cortisol increase) that can manifest as carbohydrate cravings, lethargy, poor physical/

mental performance and suboptimal recovery. Over-stimulation of insulin by fast-acting carbohydrates also can have a more insidious effect – diverting glucose into fat storage. This in turn is obviously not conducive to promoting favorable changes in body composition and metabolic health.

## Side Bar - SuperStarch

Nearly all commercially available sports and energy beverages are sugar- or cornstarch-based, emphasizing rapid absorption which is obviously anti-ketogenic. A product gaining popularity among sport enthusiasts from weekend warriors to top professional athletes is SuperStarch™, a revolutionary fuel source developed by the UCAN Company (www.generationucan.com). SuperStarch is derived from waxy maize and processed using a proprietary heat-moisture method. This process develops a unique high molecular weight product that is between 500,000 and 700,000 g/mol (compared to glucose at 180 g/mol). This results in low osmotic pressure in the gut, and slow absorption characteristics that significantly blunt spikes in blood sugar and insulin. SuperStarch has advantages over other commercially available sports drinks (and other 'me-too' waxy maize products) for use before, during and after workouts and competition. In addition to its fueling applications, an added benefit associated with regular use of SuperStarch is improved body composition.

SuperStarch was originally developed by Scottish researchers for the treatment of a rare childhood genetic disorder called glycogen storage disease, which is characterized by an impaired ability to convert glycogen to glucose in the liver. Newborn infants with glycogen storage disease need to be fed a source of carbohydrate at frequent intervals to maintain blood glucose levels, or else they risk experiencing severe hypoglycemia. SuperStarch was developed as a strategy to better manage the disease by providing extended maintenance of blood glucose. Three peer-reviewed scientific studies have confirmed that feeding SuperStarch is superior to conventional treatments in preventing hypoglycemia over extended periods of time in subjects with Glycogen Storage Disease[43, 44] and Type 1 diabetes[45]. A study was recently published in high level cyclists who ingested SuperStarch or maltodextrin before and after cycling for 2.5 hr[46]. SuperStarch blunted the initial spike in blood glucose and insulin while enhancing the breakdown and oxidation of fat during exercise. Subjects also consumed the supplements after exercise, and again the athletes showed greater use of fat during recovery.

# Chapter 7
# PROTEIN

*Necessary, But In Moderation*

**Snap Shot**

- Too little or too much protein can be problematic in the keto-adapted state.

- Aim for a protein intake between 0.6 to 1.0 grams per pound of lean body mass.

- Rather than consume large portions of meats or other protein foods, focus on small to moderate protein portions and combine them with generous portions of good sources of fat (e.g., sauces, butter, olive oil).

We can all agree that protein is the essence of your body's power. After all, protein is derived from the Greek word for primary. Our muscles, tendons, ligaments, lungs, heart, red blood cells, and enzymes are all constructed primarily of protein. However, like so many other things in life, it's important to get enough but not too much of it. In the context of both our fear of fat and now maybe cutting back on carbohydrates, deciding how much protein to eat requires a bit of diligence.

Within the nutrition and dietetics fields, most advice on protein intake is based on the recommended dietary allowance (RDA) and daily recommended intake (DRI) values. These recommendations, however, were developed for the average weight stable, unstressed individual. Add any degree of energy restriction (i.e., for weight loss) or physical or emotional stress, however, and the RDA/DRI values become inadequate. Thus consuming somewhat more protein than the recommended dietary allowance is probably justified if you are losing weight or frequently doing high stress exercise.

That said, however, significantly over-consuming protein can be problematic because some of these extra amino acids can be converted to glucose in the body, raising insulin levels, and thus driving down ketones and suppressing fat burning. Even if your goal is gaining muscle, there is a limit to how much new muscle protein can be added each day, and under most circumstances, this amount is relatively small. Over-consuming protein beyond the level that allows maximum anabolism in skeletal muscle thus puts a burden on the body to get rid of the extra nitrogen. Since protein is not a particularly efficient fuel source and for the reasons mentioned above, it therefore makes little sense to consume it in excess.

For all these reasons, we recommend aiming for an intake in the range of 0.6 to 1.0 grams per pound lean body mass. If you don't know your body composition see page 95. The table below provides a few examples of protein intake ranges for men and women with different weights and body fat contents. The key point here is that while these protein intakes are above the minimum RDA values, they are certainly not high protein intakes compared to current standards. Note also that our recommended intake ranges are pretty wide, allowing you a fair degree of flexibility in choosing your level of protein intake.

| Athlete Type | Gender | Weight (lbs) | % Body Fat | Protein grams |
|---|---|---|---|---|
| Power | Male | 200 | 15 | 102-170 |
| | Female | 150 | 20 | 72-120 |
| Endurance | Male | 165 | 10 | 89-149 |
| | Female | 120 | 15 | 61-102 |

## Post-Workout Protein

A lot of research has been dedicated to understanding how much protein you need after exercise to preserve protein synthesis and muscle protein balance. None of this work has involved keto-adapted athletes, but studies done in athletes habitually consuming moderate amounts of carbohydrate show that muscle protein balance is negative after exercise if amino acids are not provided before, during or after exercise. This has led to the common practice of consuming protein supplements after exercise, which in turn results in transient increases in muscle protein synthesis and overall positive protein balance.

It is also common practice that carbohydrates are added to protein supplements based on the belief that an increased insulin response will promote increased protein synthesis. In skeletal muscle, insulin has anabolic effects by increasing amino acid uptake and protein synthesis, but only a small amount of insulin is necessary to achieve a maximal effect[47]. The primary driver of muscle protein synthesis is not insulin, but the availability of essential amino acids, especially leucine. Thus shot-gunning a fast-acting sports drink loaded with sugar may not be the best strategy. When you weigh the trivial benefit of ingesting insulin-stimulating carbohydrates on protein balance against their potent negative effect on fat breakdown and oxidation, the net benefit comes down on the side of limiting carbohydrate intake.

**Factoid:** *When adequate protein is provided after exercise, consuming insulin-stimulating carbohydrates does not further improve the anabolic response* [48, 49].

So, what should you focus on during the post-exercise period? As we noted in Chapter 4, blood levels of leucine increase in the keto-adapted state, so sustaining a state of nutritional ketosis (by not eating carbs after exercise) will protect this benefit. There may be some benefit to including a good source of essential amino acids after resistance exercise, and especially if increased muscle mass is your goal. This does not have to be a protein supplement – your post-exercise amino acids can come from 'typical' foods. Consider a fruit smoothie made with naturally fermented yogurt, a cup of home-made meat broth, or creamed soups made from this broth. It is also a good idea to replace water and sodium loss after a workout.

**Factoid:** : *Most packaged foods list protein content per serving on the label. To determine the protein content of bulk foods, however, it helps to use 'the rule of sevens'. As a general estimate, one ounce of meat, fish, or poultry contains 7 grams of protein. A cup of fermented dairy (yogurt, buttermilk), an ounce of cheese, 2 ounces of nuts, a cup of home-made broth, and a large egg each contain about 7 grams of protein. So, for example, if your goal is to get a minimum 100 grams of protein per day, all you need to do is be sure that you include 14 of these 7-gram protein units in your daily diet.*

# Chapter 8

# FAT

*Your Most Important Fuel*

**Snap Shot**

- To maintain nutritional ketosis, as a proportion of total calories, your fat intake will need to be high (~65 to 80%).

- Since your amounts of carbohydrate and protein are locked into a relatively narrow range, the amount of fat you eat will vary depending on whether you want to lose or maintain weight.

- The fat you eat provides important fuel and therefore should emphasize the fuel sources the body prefers to burn, namely monounsaturated and saturated fats.

- Limit foods with a high proportions of the vegetable (omega-6) polyunsaturates.

- Balance your intake of omega-6 and omega-3 polyunsaturated fat.

Fat is your friend when you're consuming a low carbohydrate diet. It serves as your body's predominant fuel during both rest and exercise, and it adds flavor and satiety to your diet. Fat consumed in your food does not interfere with keto-adaption since it has virtually no impact on blood glucose or insulin levels. Since carbohydrates are necessarily limited and protein is kept within a relatively moderate range, it naturally follows that the majority of calories to support your daily activity (including training and competition) must be obtained from fat. *Therefore a key to successful keto-adaptation is figuring out ways to specifically increase your fat intake without over-consuming carbohydrate and protein*

Put another way, a lean athlete cannot survive on a diet that is simultaneously low in carbohydrate and also low in fat. Think about it – if about 20% of your daily energy comes from protein and 5-15% from carbs, where's the other 65-75% of your energy supposed to come from? The answer, of course, is 'fat'. Yes, when you are losing weight (i.e., shrinking body fat stores), some of what you burn does not need to be supplied by your diet, but this is necessarily temporary. Once you get to a stable body weight, all of your daily energy needs must be met by your dietary intake.

## How Much Fat

As you adjust your body weight and training intensity, your consumption of carbohydrates and protein will remain fairly stable despite changes in goals and activity levels, whereas how much fat you consume will be dictated by your energy demands, body weight and composition goals, and satiety. If you want to lose weight, the total amount of fat consumed will be reduced. If weight loss is not a goal, your dietary fat needs to be maintained at a level that matches your energy expenditure, thus holding your body weight stable.

This sounds like getting the right amount of fat could be complicated, but interestingly it's usually not necessary to count fat calories. Once keto-adapted, most people report that hunger and cravings are reduced. If you want to reduce your percent body fat, this increased satiety gives you the freedom to cut back a bit on how much fat you consume. If you are happy with where you are, just track your body weight or composition and use that information as well as satiety to guide you.

## The Right Types of Fat

When it comes to fat, quality is at least (if not more) important than quantity. Fats (or more specifically fatty acids) are generally classified as saturated (SFA) that contain no double bonds, monounsaturated (MUFA) that contain one double bond, and polyunsaturated (PUFA) that contain more than one double bond. The PUFA category includes the two essential fatty acid classes (omega-6 and omega-3) that humans need to consume in relatively small amounts to maintain healthy cell membranes.

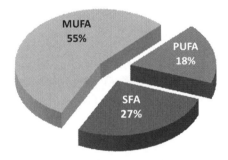

Approximate fatty acid composition of subcutaneous adipose tissue. Clearly humans prefer to store MUFA and to a lesser extent SFA. These may be the preferred fats to emphasize in the diet for fuel.

On a high fat diet, however, our requirements for these essential PUFA are met by just a small percent of our total fat intake. Thus, since the majority of fat that you consume each day is for the purpose of providing fuel (as opposed to meeting PUFA requirements), you'll want to choose fats that are easily burned. To get an idea what fats the body likes to burn, it helps to look at what our bodies choose to store in our fat cells. The fatty acids that make up the majority of triglycerides in human adipose tissue consist of SFA and MUFA. These are the fats that our bodies have selected to 'put away for a rainy day' – i.e., what we burn when there's no food. Particularly when keto-adapted (whether you are fasting or on a high fat diet), the body prefers to oxidize these fatty acids. Thus, in seeking out foods to eat, keep in mind the necessity to emphasize MUFA and SFA while keeping carbs low and consuming both protein and PUFA in moderation.

*Factoid: A 50:50 mixture of butter and olive oil approximates the composition of triglycerides typically found in human body fat.*

You might be thinking that these guys are inappropriately encouraging consumption of saturated fats, given all the hype about it being related to heart disease. On careful inspection of the scientific literature, however, the widespread belief that dietary saturated fat is harmful turns out to be an out-dated paradigm based upon flawed reasoning.

Yes, we know that this looks like an outrageous statement. So here is a brief summary of the details. Current evidence shows no association between dietary saturated fat intake and cardiovascular disease (CVD)[50, 51]. There is, however, a consistent pattern of increased risk for CVD[52-55] and diabetes[56-58] associated with increased amounts of saturated fat circulating in the blood. It is a common mistake for people to assume that your intake of saturates is what determines your blood level of this much maligned nutrient, but this is incorrect. Particularly in the keto-adapted state, fat is being burned at a much higher rate, and this is particularly true for saturated fat. In two recently published studies we showed that a low carbohydrate, high fat diet significantly decreased circulating levels of saturated fat[23, 59]. It's hard to imagine how dietary saturated fat can be problematic when it is promptly burned to carbon dioxide and water.

## Omega-3 and Omega-6 Fats

Among the polyunsaturated fats, there are two essential classes called omega-3 and omega-6. The actual human requirement for these two forms of PUFA is low – about ~1% of daily energy from each of these two classes. Most Americans consume about ten times the amount of omega-6 they need due to frequent intake of soy, corn, cottonseed, peanut, sunflower, and safflower oils. By contrast, many of us barely meet our daily minimum 1% for omega-3. Furthermore, because a high omega-6 intake can interfere with omega-3 metabolism, this disparity between omega-6 and omega-3 intakes throws off the balance between these two competing classes of essential fats, making our marginal omega-3 intake worse.

The clinical importance of consuming a lower omega-6 to omega-3 ratio is well established[60], but there are additional reasons why athletes may benefit. Omega-6 fats are more strongly associated with inflammation than omega-3 fats. Increasing omega-3 status consistently leads to lower levels of inflammation, and it also has a potent effect on lowering fat levels (triglycerides) in the blood. In addition to being linked to many chronic disease states, chronic elevations in inflammation can impair recovery from exercise, compromise adaptations to training, and increased risk of injury.

*Factoid:* *Peak aerobic power, also called* $VO_2max$, *is negatively associated with biomarkers of inflammation like interleukin-6 and c-reactive protein[61]. This implies that reducing inflammation facilitates cellular energy metabolism and increases work performance.*

## Side Bar – Emerging Omega-3 Fat Research Relevant to Athletes

Studies show that increasing membrane omega-3 fatty acids enhances insulin sensitivity, promotes fat burning in muscles, and inhibits fat storage. Recent work indicates that omega-3 fats may regulate muscle growth and help during periods of muscle disuse by slowing muscle and bone loss[62]. This could be applicable for athletes during breaks in training or layoffs due to injury where muscle loss could be significant. Omega-3 fats have also been shown to augment blood flow to muscles during exercise[63]. Moreover, omega-3's in combination with exercise were recently shown to maximize fat loss[64]. In

addition, subjects supplemented with fish oil decreased blood triglycerides, increased high density lipoprotein cholesterol, and improved
the functioning of blood vessels. According to recent work, omega-3s
were shown to decrease muscle soreness and swelling and increase
range of motion after damaging exercise[65].

## Why Worry About Too Much Omega-6 PUFA?

Back in the day when Steve did his study with the bike racers on the ketogenic diet, they had to measure precisely how much of each nutrient his
subjects were eating. That limited him to just five menu items from which
his subjects could choose each day. Three of these were composed principally of animal fats and two used soybean oil mayonnaise as their fat source.
Within a week or two of starting the high fat diet, most of the subjects developed a strong distaste for the mayonnaise-based meals. Opening a new
container and then switching brands of mayonnaise didn't help. Nobody
actually got sick eating these tuna salad or chicken salad entrees – they just
said that they didn't feel completely well after eating them.

Out of curiosity, Steve put himself on a ketogenic diet for a month and
fed himself most of his fat intake overnight via a tiny feeding tube in his
stomach (so taste wasn't an issue). Within 3 days of feeding himself 1500
Calories of either soybean or corn oil nightly, he developed quite prominent nausea and gastro-intestinal upset. However when he fed himself
the same amount of calories as olive oil for two straight weeks, he had no
such symptoms. In between testing these different oils via the feeding
tube, Steve maintained nutritional ketosis and met his full calorie needs
by eating mostly animal fats, again without symptoms.

The take-away message from this is that the human system doesn't seem
to tolerate a high fat diet prepared from high omega-6 oils (like soy and
corn oils), but does just fine on one consisting mostly of monounsaturated and saturated fats (e.g., olive oil and animal fats). This doesn't mean
you can't eat mayo, just find one made from olive or canola oil or make
your own. And please, don't be fooled by the ag-industry advertising that

touts high PUFA oils as being heart healthy. While this message might have some validity for someone eating a very low fat diet, at the high fat end of the dietary fat spectrum, it is completely invalid (if not dangerous).

We've met numerous people who tried a low-carbohydrate, high-fat diet and promptly quit it, saying : "I couldn't handle eating all that fat!" When queried, they often noted that they'd tried to "eat healthy" by avoiding animal fats, which means they probably were eating way too much omega-6 PUFA. This is all too easy to do, as most mayonnaise, salad dressings, and marinades (whether bargain brands or named after boxers or movie stars) are based on lowly soybean oil. Removing most of this high omega-6 vegetable oil from your intake will remove a major barrier to feeling well and functioning well, and thus being able to sustain your ketogenic diet long-term.

## Practical Guidelines on Consuming Fat

Foods rich in fat contain a mix of different fatty acids, and it will serve you well to have a good understanding of the ones that contain primarily saturated and monounsaturated fat. It also helps to have knowledge of how to prepare and incorporate them into your diet.

*Fats and Oils* Purely fat-containing foods vary widely in their composition. The best oils to use are those that are low in PUFA, such as olive, canola, 'high oleic' safflower, coconut and palm. Steer clear of corn, soybean, cottonseed, peanut, and safflower, as well as margarines and mayonnaise made with any of these oils. Butter and fat from beef (tallow) or pork (lard) are also excellent choices, both as they occur in natural foods and as fats added in cooking. Since they contain practically zero carbohydrates, use them liberally. Be creative and try to use these fats/oils with as many foods as possible (e.g., salad dressings, marinades, sautéing, stir-frying).

*Other Fat-Containing Foods.* Most other fat-containing foods that also contain protein and a few carbs are naturally low in PUFA so they can be used regularly. Animal fats such as those in meats, eggs, and dairy are relatively low in PUFA and good sources of SFA and MUFA. Other good sources of fat are olives, avocados, heavy cream, sour cream, nuts, seeds, and cheese.

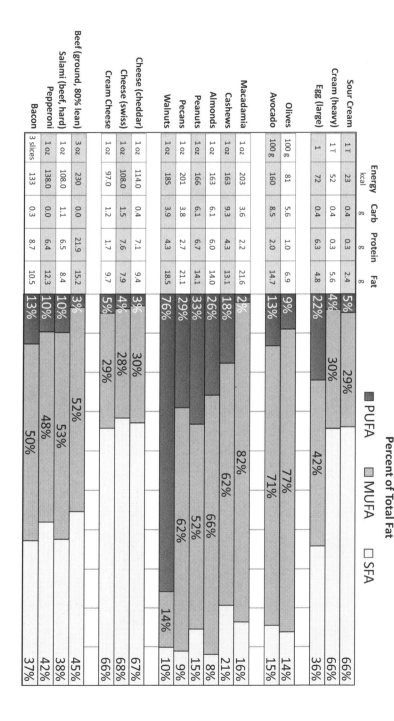

**Percent of Total Fat** — ■ PUFA  ▨ MUFA  ☐ SFA

| | | Energy kcal | Carb g | Protein g | Fat g | PUFA | MUFA | SFA |
|---|---|---|---|---|---|---|---|---|
| Sour Cream | 1 T | 23 | 0.4 | 0.3 | 2.4 | 5% | 29% | 66% |
| Cream (heavy) | 1 T | 52 | 0.4 | 0.3 | 5.6 | 4% | 30% | 66% |
| Egg (large) | 1 | 72 | 0.4 | 6.3 | 4.8 | 22% | 42% | 36% |
| Olives | 100 g | 81 | 5.6 | 1.0 | 6.9 | 9% | 77% | 14% |
| Avocado | 100 g | 160 | 8.5 | 2.0 | 14.7 | 13% | 71% | 15% |
| Macadamia | 1 oz | 203 | 3.6 | 2.2 | 21.6 | 2% | 82% | 16% |
| Cashews | 1 oz | 163 | 9.3 | 4.3 | 13.1 | 18% | 62% | 21% |
| Almonds | 1 oz | 163 | 6.1 | 6.0 | 14.0 | 26% | 66% | 8% |
| Peanuts | 1 oz | 166 | 6.1 | 6.7 | 14.1 | 33% | 52% | 15% |
| Pecans | 1 oz | 201 | 3.8 | 2.7 | 21.1 | 29% | 62% | 9% |
| Walnuts | 1 oz | 185 | 3.9 | 4.3 | 18.5 | 76% | 14% | 10% |
| Cream Cheese | 1 oz | 97.0 | 1.2 | 1.7 | 9.7 | 5% | 29% | 66% |
| Cheese (swiss) | 1 oz | 108.0 | 1.5 | 7.6 | 7.9 | 4% | 28% | 68% |
| Cheese (cheddar) | 1 oz | 114.0 | 0.4 | 7.1 | 9.4 | 3% | 30% | 67% |
| Beef (ground, 80% lean) | 3 oz | 230 | 0.0 | 21.9 | 15.2 | 3% | 52% | 45% |
| Salami (beef, hard) | 1 oz | 108.0 | 1.1 | 6.5 | 8.4 | 10% | 53% | 38% |
| Pepperoni | 1 oz | 138.0 | 0.0 | 6.4 | 12.3 | 10% | 48% | 42% |
| Bacon | 3 slices | 133 | 0.3 | 8.7 | 10.5 | 13% | 50% | 37% |

| | | Energy kcal | Carb g | Protein g | Fat g | Percent of Total Fat ■ PUFA ▨ MUFA ☐ SFA | | |
|---|---|---|---|---|---|---|---|---|
| Oil (coconut) | 1 T | 117 | 0.0 | 0.0 | 13.6 | 2% | 6% | 92% |
| Butter | 1 T | 102 | 0.0 | 0.1 | 11.5 | 4% | 28% | 68% |
| Beef Tallow | 1 T | 115 | 0.0 | 0.0 | 12.8 | 4% | 44% | 52% |
| Oil (palm) | 1 T | 120 | 0.0 | 0.0 | 13.6 | 10% | 39% | 52% |
| Oil (olive) | 1 T | 119 | 0.0 | 0.0 | 13.5 | 11% | 75% | 14% |
| Lard | 1 T | 115 | 0.0 | 0.0 | 12.8 | 12% | 47% | 41% |
| Oil (safflower, high oleic) | 1 T | 120 | 0.0 | 0.0 | 13.6 | 13% | 79% | 8% |
| Oil (canola) | 1 T | 124 | 0.0 | 0.0 | 14.0 | 28% | 64% | 7% |
| Oil (peanut) | 1 T | 119 | 0.0 | 0.0 | 13.5 | 34% | 49% | 18% |
| Oil (corn) | 1 T | 120 | 0.0 | 0.0 | 13.6 | 57% | 29% | 14% |
| Oil (soybean) | 1 T | 120 | 0.0 | 0.0 | 13.6 | 60% | 24% | 16% |
| Oil (safflower) | 1 T | 120 | 0.0 | 0.0 | 13.6 | 78% | 15% | 6% |

## Practical Guidelines for Omega-3 Intake

As noted above, although there is wide variability across individuals, most Americans barely meet the minimum requirement for omega-3 fatty acids, let alone achieve an optimal level of intake. The minimum dose to start is 500 mg of EPA plus DHA per day, which is equivalent to about one serving of fatty fish every other day. A more optimal dose for most people may be closer to 1 gram per day of EPA and DHA. If you are at high risk of heart disease, stroke or inflammatory condition, then 2 grams per day may result in better effects.

Fish from cold water are the richest source of the main omega-3 fats (EPA [20:5] and DHA [22:6]) that we need to maintain healthy membranes. Good sources of these fatty acids are salmon, tuna, sardines, and herring. Ideally consume them 2-3 times per week. Alpha-linolenate (18:3) is an omega-3 precursor to EPA/DHA found in flax and canola oil and to a lesser extent in some nuts like walnuts and almonds, but the conversion to EPA and DHA in humans is not efficient. Thus if you don't eat cold water fish, supplementation with a source of EPA and DHA may be prudent.

A readily available alternative to eating fish or fish oil capsules is omega-3 eggs. These are produced by feeding hens a diet rich in omega-3 fats, resulting in 100-150 mg of EPA + DHA per egg. Thus two of these omega-3 eggs get you close to the minimum daily dose without the need to eat fish.

The response to omega-3 rich foods or fish oil supplementation varies between people, and some individuals require higher doses to achieve physiological effects. Ideally we encourage you to test your blood or cheek cells for EPA and DHA content (http://www.omega3test.com/) (see Chapter 10).

*Factoid: Usually DHA is derived from cold water fish, but a new method is available where DHA is produced from microalgae with no EPA (Neuromins™ by Martek). For those readers who are vegan vegetarians, do not like the taste of fish, or who find fish oil capsules unacceptable, DHA derived from microalgae at a minimum dose of 200 mg per day is a viable option.*

# Chapter 9

# FLUID AND MINERAL MANAGEMENT

*Why Micronutrients Can Have A Macro-Effect*

**Snap Shot**

- Low carbohydrate diets increase the loss of sodium and water by the kidneys.

- Failure to adequately replace sodium adversely affects potassium balance and has several negative effects (e.g., fatigue, fainting, headache, loss of lean mass).

- The easiest solution is to consume an extra 1-2 grams of sodium per day in the form of 2 bouillon cubes (or home-made broth).

- Most muscle cramps are due to magnesium depletion in cells.

- Adequate magnesium intake helps prevent cramps.

- A 20 day course of slow-release magnesium supplementation effectively treats most muscle cramps.

- Dietary magnesium and potassium (as well as other micronutrients) can be increased by appropriate preparation of meats and vegetables.

Most diet books that bother to explain metabolism at all focus on protein (to build or maintain structure), plus some combination of fats and carbohydrates for fuel. Minerals aren't sexy, so why waste the paper (or electrons if you are reading this as an e-book) talking about them? To answer this, think of proteins as bricks used to build a wall. Now think of minerals as the mortar that keeps the bricks together. Or if you prefer a car analogy think of fat as the high octane gas powering your engine (which it does when you are keto-adapted). Now think of minerals as the transmission that connects your engine to the wheels.

Low carbohydrate diets change how your body uses minerals, particularly sodium and potassium. Other commonly neglected minerals such as magnesium and zinc are just as important whichever diet you choose, and ignoring them can impair your well-being and function. If you are interested in optimizing your ability to function, ignore this chapter at your peril.

## Sodium

There are two classes of athletes: the smart ones who understand that they need to manage their sodium intake, and the others who don't. Most athletes sweat, and sweat contains salt. Both sweat and blood taste 'salty', because both contain an appreciable amount sodium. The only place inside your body where you find much sodium is in the blood, so if you run short of it, there's not much 'on reserve' elsewhere in the body. Thus, if you don't have enough sodium, your circulation (aka circulating blood volume) has to shrink. Sweat too much and your body runs short of sodium, and this forces it to shrink your blood volume to keep serum sodium concentration in the normal range. Shrink your circulating volume too much and you pass out.

Thus salt is a critically important nutrient for athletes, and this is especially true on a low carbohydrate diet. When carbohydrates are restricted the body changes from retaining both water and salt to discarding them. Because of this fundamental shift in mineral management, it's not uncommon for people to lose 4-5 pounds of water weight during the first week of a low carbohydrate diet. Typically, only half of that first week's weight loss is from fat and the other half is due to salt loss along with its associated water. If some of that salt is not replaced, however, blood flow may be impaired and the body over-reacts in its quest for salt. This primarily happens in the kidneys, which try to compensate by wasting potassium (i.e., kidney cells give up potassium in exchange for retaining sodium), leading to a negative potassium balance.

What does all this mean? The loss of water and salt can reduce plasma volume and make you feel sluggish and compromise your ability to perform outdoors in the heat or in the weight room. As a result, some people get headaches and feel faint. This state of salt depletion causes a compensatory loss of potassium, which has a negative impact on muscle mass since potassium is a necessary co-factor in building and maintaining skeletal muscle. The easy solution is to routinely take 1-2 grams of sodium per day in the form of 2 bouillon cubes (or home-made broth). Some bouillon cubes contain less than 1 gram sodium so be sure to check. On days that you exercise, be sure to take one dose of broth or bouillon 30 minutes before your workout.

*Factoid:* *The average American currently consumes between 5 and 10 grams of sodium per day. In the context of a high carbohydrate intake (which programs the kidneys to retain sodium), this is way too high of a sodium (salt) intake. But since cutting carb intake fundamentally changes how the kidneys handle salt, it is not clear that the common mantra "the less salt, the better" is correct when you are on ketogenic diet.*

Because we've all heard this 'reduce the salt' mantra, when we 'go on a diet', we naturally tend to cut back in sodium as well as calories. It's the specific combination of severely reduced sodium intake (under 3 grams per day) along with a ketogenic diet that causes the problems we are talking about here (sometimes called the 'Atkins Flu'). By adding back 2 grams of sodium as broth or bouillon, and timing these before exercise or heat stress, all of these problems are banished. Since a low carbohydrate diet speeds salt excretion by the kidneys, and since this adds up to a total sodium intake that's still less than 5 grams per day (well below the American average), this is fully safe in this context.

We understand that this is a tough sell when all doctors, dietitians, and most of the general public has accepted the uniform message that salt is bad. But think about the alternative: if your low carb, low salt diet makes you feel lousy all the time and you can't exercise without feeling faint or passing out, the problems with this diet begin to outweigh its benefits. Whether the potential benefit of your low carb lifestyle is putting type-2 diabetes into remission or running a pain-free marathon, neither will happen until you get this salt issue resolved.

So unless you have very high blood pressure, try adding back a couple servings of broth per day. If you are worried about your blood pressure, get a cuff and measure it to be sure it stays normal (which it usually does on a ketogenic diet). The simple hard truth is that if you can't get your salt intake properly adjusted to prevent the 'Atkins Flu', you won't stay on a ketogenic diet and be able to reap its benefits for the long run (pun intended).

## Potassium

When someone says 'potassium', dietitians instantly think 'orange juice' and 'bananas', neither of which is much help if you want to stay keto-adapted. Few dietitians think of meats and low starch vegetables as excellent sources of potassium, but they are. There's as much potassium in 4 oz of meat as in a medium banana or 8 oz of orange juice. However the Achilles heel of meat and vegetables as potassium sources is how they are prepared. Boil either one and much of the potassium is lost in the broth. If you grill your meat to medium well done, much of the potassium leaves with the drippings.

The obvious solution is to not discard 'the solution' (i.e., the potassium-containing broth and drippings). Cook meats so the drippings aren't lost and steam or sauté vegetables rather than boiling them. Enjoy your daily allotments of berries, nuts, and seeds, which all contain appreciable amounts of potassium. Most importantly, consider making your own broth. A chicken carcass boiled for a few hours gives up much of its potassium to the broth, as is true for beef bones and scraps as well. Add all of these together and a well-formulated low carbohydrate diet turns out to be richly endowed with potassium, one of the key minerals keeping you upright and functioning well.

## Hydration

Because of the fluid shift associated with nutritional ketosis, an athlete starting a long event or workout begins with less total fluid on board then if s/he had prepared by eating a high carb diet. It's also important to understand that during the first 5-10 minutes of exercise, there is a normal expansion of the circulation (aka plasma volume). These two factors can leave the low-carb athlete feeling inappropriately thirsty and sluggish in the first 5-15 minutes of hard exercise. The solution is to drink 1-2 cups (250-500 ml) of water about 5 minutes before starting – long enough for most of it to be absorbed but too soon for your kidneys to start clearing it. Once exercising, kidney blood flow goes way down, so that initial priming dose of water is retained and supports the early exercise plasma volume expansion.

During prolonged events, maintain your hydration with water or other low carbohydrate beverages. If you are sweating profusely for a number of hours, consider adding back some salt as broth or bouillon to compensate for the sodium you have lost in your sweat.

## Magnesium

If you have ever been brought up short in training or in competition by a muscle cramp, you need to read this section. Ask most coaches or most doctors what causes muscle cramps and you will hear: a) dehydration, b) not enough potassium, or c) not enough calcium. Only a few percent of either group will tell you that you've got a magnesium problem, but those few are usually right.

Magnesium resides inside our cells. There is very little of it in serum, so blood tests for this mineral can't tell us if we are okay or not. As a result, doctors (who rely on blood tests for most assays), are generally clueless about magnesium.

Magnesium calms muscles (including the heart), nerves, and the brain. When magnesium levels fall in these organs, they get 'twitchy'. Stress them with intense exercise, sleep deprivation, or not enough fuel, and twitchy becomes spasm (aka cramping). If a muscle cramps, you stop using it. If your brain cramps, you have a seizure. If your heart cramps, you die. Luckily, these last two signs of magnesium depletion are rare. But we've all seen hundreds of athletes cramp a muscle, but seldom do they know why.

Because magnesium is critical for muscle function, there's quite a bit of it in meat. But if you boil or process that meat (like make it into a hot dog), most of the magnesium is lost. Similarly, magnesium is the mineral at the core of chlorophyll – the green stuff that makes photosynthesis (and thus all sunlight-powered life) possible. The darker green the vegetable, the more magnesium it contains. But if you boil it until it's mushy, when you throw away the water, you throw away much of the magnesium.

So here's the key to getting enough magnesium from your diet. When you cook meat, capture the drippings and add it back as sauce. If you boil meat or bones, drink the broth or reduce it to make sauce. Steam vegetables rather than boiling them, and cook them until they are 'al dente' (to the tooth) rather than soft enough to eat without teeth. Do all of these things routinely and you'll probably get enough magnesium from your diet without supplements.

But if you have frequent muscle cramps, your first order of business is to make them stop. Cramps during or after exercise, or even at night, are a sign that your body has a major magnesium deficit. So here's the shortcut to ending most night-time or post-exercise muscle cramps. Take 3 slow-release magnesium tablets daily for 20 days. The proprietary brand-name product is 'Slow-Mag' ™, but there are a number of equally effective generics now available at a fraction of the brand-name price (e.g., Mag-64™ or

Mag-Delay™). Most people's cramps cease within 2 weeks of starting this dose of Slow-Mag™, but you should continue to take the full 20-day course (60 tablets per bottle at 3 per day lasts 20 days). If the cramps return later, do it again, but after re-doing those first 20 days at 3 pills per day, then continue taking one pill per day. If despite this, the cramps return, take 2 pills per day for perpetuity. Most people can be titrated to remain cramp-free by this method.

Why, you may ask, do you need to use a more expensive slow-release preparation like Slow-Mag™ or even its generic equivalent? The answer is that the more common magnesium oxide (such as Milk of Magnesia™) preparations cause diarrhea – they pass right through you with relatively little being absorbed. And magnesium gluconate (another popular magnesium supplement) is mostly 'gluconate' (a form of sugar), so those big pills don't actually contain as much magnesium as they do carbohydrate.

WARNING: The only significant risk to taking oral magnesium supplements is for people with severe kidney failure. If you have a history of kidney problems or known loss of kidney function, check with your doctor before taking Slow-Mag™ or its generic equivalents.

## Zinc

Most people, including athletes, don't need to worry about getting enough zinc; but zinc is absolutely required for growth, protein synthesis (building muscle), healing, and your body's defense against infection. So if you are one of the minority who has a zinc problem, it is definitely going to affect your well-being and physical performance.

Signs of zinc deficiency are severe dry skin, horizontal depressions across the fingernails, and recurrent skin warts (e.g., plantar warts on the soles of the feet). Zinc deficiency is not uncommon in the elderly due to poor diet and reduced ability to absorb this mineral from the small intestine. In younger people, however, there are two causes of zinc inadequacy. The first is rapid growth during adolescence, particularly if the diet is composed of highly refined foods. The other cause is iron

– specifically people who are given iron pills by their doctor due to low blood hemoglobin (anemia).

Anemia is justifiably a major concern in athletes, because hemoglobin (the iron-containing protein that makes blood red) is the stuff that carries oxygen in your blood. If you have too little of it, your performance is impaired. Thus doctors are prone to give athletes iron if their blood hemoglobin is even slightly on the low side. The connection between iron and zinc is that both are trace minerals that are absorbed by the same mechanism in the small intestine. This means that taking lots of iron for months at a time blocks absorption of zinc, even if there is plenty of zinc in your diet.

The solution to this problem is simple. If you are on iron for anemia, take it as directed by your doctor but ask his/her permission to take it only EVERY OTHER MONTH. In the intervening months, take 50 mg of zinc (preferable as chloride rather than gluconate) once per day. Both of these zinc supplements are available over-the-counter. This won't work if you try to take the iron and zinc together, because at these doses they compete and block each other's absorption. And don't worry about skipping iron every other month, because if you are zinc depleted, all the iron in the world may not cure your anemia[66].

WARNING: Even if you are not on iron pills, if you choose to take zinc as recommended above, take it for only 30 days at a time, and wait at least another 30 days before taking it again. Staying on this dose of zinc continuously can cause you to come up short on other trace minerals like iron and copper.

## Summary

The key information in this chapter specific to low carbohydrate diets is that you need a consistent, <u>modest</u> intake of salt (sodium) along with a consistent intake of potassium when you are keto-adapted. Everyone who follows a low carbohydrate life-style needs to heed this caution, because not doing so will dependably lead to fatigue, light-headedness, and impaired physical performance.

Our advice concerning magnesium and zinc has nothing to do specifically with a low carbohydrate diet. Nonetheless, if you had a problem with either one of these minerals before you transition to a low carb diet, it's not going to go away just because you've reduced your dietary carbohydrates. Whatever diet you are on, magnesium or zinc inadequacies will slow you down, so we've offered you our solutions to both. Even if you don't have a problem with these minerals yourself, chances are that you know someone who does. If their reaction to resolving these problems is anything like what we get from our patients, you'll be a hero for passing this message along.

# Chapter 10

# PERSONALIZATION

*Finding Your Ketone Zone And More*

## Snap Shot

- To achieve optimal fuel flow during keto-adaptation you should aim for blood ketone levels between 0.5 and 3.0 millimolar.

- The most practical, accurate, and fast way to test ketones is to use a hand held monitor that measures BOHB in a drop of blood.

- Several factors act to increase blood ketones including restricting carbohydrate, keeping protein moderate, exercise, and ingestion of medium chain triglycerides found in butter and coconut oil.

- Monitoring body composition using dual-energy x-ray absorptiometry (DXA) is the most accurate way to assess changes in whole body and regional fat, lean, and bone mass.

- Measuring specific blood fatty acids (and perhaps noninvasively in cheek cells) provides individualized guidance on carbohydrate intake, omega 3 status, and overtraining.

For the past century, the nutrition establishment has been striving to find the one perfect diet for everyone. For anyone walking down the street with their eyes open, or trying to comfortably fit between two other adults in airline seating, this 'unified dietary hypothesis' obviously has been an abject failure. Clearly this process had led us to a diet that is right for a third of us but wrong for the other two thirds. Equally as clearly, finding which diet – and specifically how much carbohydrate – is right for you requires a credible system of personalized guidance. The science of personalized testing is rapidly emerging from the research laboratory and into your home and gym. Here are a few tools that you can employ to chart your individual course to improved health and function.

## The Ketone Zone

In order to experience the full spectrum of metabolic benefits associated with keto-adaptation, it is necessary to restrict your carbohydrate and consume moderate protein to allow blood ketones to come up into the desirable range. In a healthy person normally consuming carbohydrate-rich foods (>100 grams/day), blood ketone levels (usually consisting of a 4-to-1 ratio of BOHB to AcAc) rarely exceed 0.2 millimolar. As carbohydrates are decreased to below 50 grams per day and protein is not consumed in excess, most people will produce ketone levels >0.5 millimolar. In Steve's study of competitive cyclists riding 100-200 miles per week and consuming a very low carbohydrate (less than 10 grams per day) ketogenic diet for 4 weeks, they had resting levels of BOHB between 1.5 and 2.5 millimolar[6] and in overweight women consuming a hypocaloric ketogenic diet the levels were about the same or even higher[7].

There are a number of factors that can be used to determine the best level of blood ketones. One would be that level required to replace much of the brain's glucose use with ketones. A second criterion would be the blood ketone concentration that reduces the body's oxidation of the essential amino acid leucine. We know that this occurs because blood leucine levels rose sharply in Steve's bike racers when they became keto-adapted, and also because another study showed that BOHB infused intravenously reduced leucine oxidation and increased the body's rate of protein synthesis[67]. Taking these factors in combination, a therapeutic range of blood ketone levels for an athlete starts at 0.5 millimolar BOHB at the lower end and improves up to 3.0 millimolar. There do not appear to be any benefits to pushing blood ketones higher than 3 millimolar, which is about as high as most people get eating a well-formulated ketogenic diet.

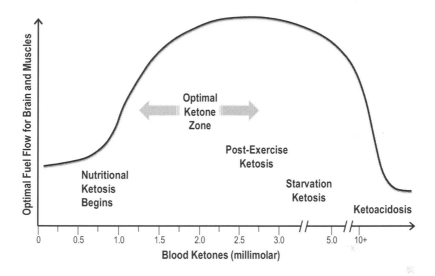

## Monitoring Ketones

So how do you know if your ketones are in the optimum range? A credible method to determine if you are in the right ketone zone will provide you with essential feedback on how you are responding to your diet. Ketones have typically been measured in urine, blood, or breath; and each has its advantages and disadvantages.

Urine is the most common method used to track ketosis because it is the cheapest and easiest test. Reagent strips (dipsticks) containing sodium nitroprusside dipped in urine change to varying shades of purple in proportion to the level of AcAc (and to some extent acetone) present. The degree of color change provides a semi-quantitative measure of ketone concentration in urine, but this test has been found to inaccurately reflect actual blood ketone concentrations in several studies[68]. This is because keto-adaptation involves complex changes in the way the kidneys filter blood and thus excretion of ketones. As a result, urine ketones may decrease even as blood values stay in the desirable range. Therefore, although this method is practical and relatively inexpensive, its results should be viewed with a considerable degree of caution.

Blood tests for ketones are more definitive since they measure the concentration of BOHB, AcAc, or both, where it is most important – directly in your circulation. This can be done by having your blood drawn (usually requiring a doctor's order) and sending it to an expensive clinical laboratory. A faster and more practical method is available by means of home blood testing devices that assess BOHB in blood obtained from a finger stick. For example, Precision Xtra® (Abbott Diabetes Care, Inc) and Nova Max® Plus (Nova Biomedical) are reasonably priced devices (~$20) available 'over-the-counter' that can test for levels of BOHB and glucose in a matter of seconds. However, reagent strips for BOHB are relatively expensive (~$3 to 5 per strip) if purchased at retail drug stores. On eBay, however, it is possible to buy these same blood ketone strips for $1-2 each.

Even this reduced price may seem like a lot to pay to test your individual response, but this investment for a few months of testing provides valuable feedback on whether you are in the right ketone zone. Think about it: what if minor changes in your intake of carbs and/or protein could boost you from 0.4 millimolar BOHB to 2.0 millimolar? At this lower level, ketones are doing little to feed your brain or help you build muscle, whereas at or above 2.0 millimolar BOHB, both would be working strongly in your favor. Is this worth paying $20 for the test meter, $2 per test, and pricking your fingertip once per day for a month or two? Based upon our experience working with many people, we think that the answer is "yes".

There are also devices in development that will test the concentration of acetone in breath; which in turn has been shown to correlate well with blood ketones[69]. This breath test is better than urine ketones because the lungs don't filter the acetone. In all likelihood, one or more breath ketone analyzers will be commercially available soon. When they are, you'll have a hand-held device that you can blow into and know your body's ketone level in less than a minute. What will this device save you? The cost per test likely will be about the same as the Abbott device, so all you'll save with a breath analyzer would be biting you lip and pricking a fingertip. The current bottom line: don't hold your breath waiting for the breath analyzer.

## Factors Impacting Ketone Production

A number of factors impact blood ketones, and there is wide variability between people. If you are struggling getting into ketosis or wondering why your levels vary from one reading to the next, it helps to have an understanding of the major factors impacting blood ketone levels.

*Carbohydrate.* Nearly all the regulatory steps involved in production of ketones are inhibited by insulin, so ketone levels are exquisitely sensitive to carbohydrate ingestion. There is no one magic number for carbohydrate intake that optimizes ketone production for every individual. That said, as a ball-park guess, we have found that 50 grams per day is a good target for most people to stay below if they want to keep plasma ketones above 0.5 millimolar. Given the range in peoples' responses, however, some individuals need to stay under 30 grams whereas others can consume as much as 100 grams per day of total carbs and still remain in nutritional ketosis. It is this variability that argues in favor of testing your blood ketones daily for the first few months of a low carbohydrate diet until you know how to keep yourself in the optimum ketone zone of the diagram above.

*Protein.* Another important nutritional factor that impacts ketone production is protein intake. At the same low level of carbohydrate, increasing the amountof protein to fat in your diet will impede ketone production. This is because a little over half of the amino acids in protein are converted to glucose in the body, producing an anti-ketogenic effect. This is not a trivial point for athletes since high protein diets and the use of protein shakes before and after workouts are commonly encouraged. However, on a low carbohydrate diet the proper balance of protein and fat needs to be carefully adjusted in order to achieve optimal fat burning.

Again, this is an argument to get a hand held ketone meter and test your blood BOHB levels until you've characterized your personal response.

*Exercise.* If you test your blood ketones after exercise, they usually increase between 0.25 - 0.5 millimolar indicating effective stimulation of fat burning. Ketone levels increase sharply during the 1-2 hours after exercise due to increased hepatic delivery of fatty acids and greater rates of fat oxidation. This will be attenuated if carbohydrate is consumed after exercise, and completely blunted if high amounts of the amino acid alanine are ingested[70]. The anti-ketogenic nature of alanine may be related to its ability to increase mitochondrial oxaloacetate levels and thereby decrease acetyl CoA and production of ketones[71]. Since this rise in ketones after exercise is beneficial, it is better to avoid foods or supplements that prevent or suppress it.

**Factoid:** *The rise in blood ketones after exercise, the so-called 'Courtice-Douglas effect', was first documented in 1936[72]. After a marathon, even an athlete who has carbohydrate loaded and consumed sugars along the course may have blood ketones up to 0.5 mM when crossing the finish line. However getting ketones up to this threshold level by running for a few hours does not achieve keto-adaptation – that still takes a couple of weeks of sustained low carb intake.*

*Time of Day.* In people adapted to a very low carbohydrate diet, there also appears to be a small diurnal variation in ketones with lowest levels observed in the morning after an overnight fast with levels gradually increasing over the day. In children consuming a ketogenic diet for management of seizures, both blood BOHB and AcAc gradually increased from morning to mid afternoon on the order of 25%[73]. Other work in healthy adults has shown gradual increases in blood ketones over the course of the day and more rapid increases after meals low in carbohydrate and high in fat[69, 73].

*Medium Chain Triglycerides.* Unlike most of the fats we eat (i.e., the long-chain triglycerides [LCT] having between 14 and 18 carbons per fatty acid), medium-chain triglycerides (MCT) are made from smaller fatty acids that range between 6-12 carbons in length. In respect to their metabolism, MCT have three very important distinctions from LCT. First, they are absorbed much more quickly. Second, MCT don't get stored in fat cells, so once consumed, they need to be processed immediately. Third, MCT are not dependent on the same regulatory factors that control LCT entry into cells and mitochondria; so MCT are promptly oxidized in muscle cells or used by the liver to make ketones. Thus, depending on the dose, ingestion of MCTs can result in rapid elevation of ketones.

Natural sources of MCT are dairy fats (e.g., butter and cream) and coconut oil, so you may find your ketones go up more after ingestion of these foods. About 10-15% of the fat in butter consists of MCTs, and about two-thirds of the fat in coconut oil is MCT (mainly lauric acid [12:0]). You can also purchase MCT oil as a supplement. Ingestion of MCT oil will result in significant ketosis even if consumed with carbohydrates, although this MCT-induced ketone production may not be associated with the full spectrum of metabolic benefits associated with carbohydrate-restricted keto-adaptation. Thus, we do not encourage use of MCT oil. That said, however, neither do we discourage consuming foods that naturally contain MCT.

## Body Composition

Beyond body weight, it is helpful to know how those pounds are divided between fat and lean tissue (aka body composition). There are many body composition techniques available in clinics and gyms, but most of them are too inaccurate to be useful for individual testing (as opposed to measuring average changes in a large group). Among the tests available, dual-energy x-ray absorptiometry (DXA) is the most accurate and provides additional information beyond other common body composition methods. Other tests you may have access to at your gym such as skin folds, Bod Pod, and bioelectrical impedance are cheaper, but their re-

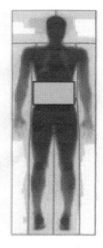

sults can vary widely due to changes in hydration, body temperature, and skin moisture. A DXA scan provides information about whole body and regional lean and fat tissue, as well as bone mass. For example, specific information can be provided about fat content in the abdominal area.

We encourage you to track your progress by measuring body composition. At the least, we highly recommend you consider having a DXA done after 3 or 6 months of keto-adaptation. Even better would be to obtain a baseline body composition study before you start a low carb diet and then after 3-6 months so you can track your reduction in body fat resulting from reduced insulin and improved access to body fat reserves for energy.

In our experience the cost of a DXA ranges between $75 and $200 and provides quantitative information on whole body and regional fat mass, lean body mass, and bone mineral density. To obtain this test, it's worth doing some investigative work to find a location near you. DXAs are available in most hospitals, clinics, and some commercial testing centers. You can try searching online using key words "body composition" and "DXA" and "major city, state near you". When you schedule a DXA test, state clearly that you are looking for body fat and lean body mass results as well as bone density.

What you can expect to get from before and after DXA studies are accurate assessments of changes in total body fat, regional body fat, and lean body mass. If you don't see much weight loss, but your DXA studies show increased lean tissue, you can be confident that you are trading fat pounds for lean pounds. If you start with extra lean tissue and lose some of it commensurate with major weight loss, that's potentially appropriate. In contrast, however, if you start out being overweight but relatively low in lean body mass, you need to jealously guard your lean tissue by maintaining adequate protein intake. In this case, you would want to see your lean body mass increase after a few months on a well-formulated ketogenic diet; and if not, adjust protein and minerals to allow that to happen.

## Future Personalized Methods on the Horizon (Stay Tuned)

*POA Testing From Cheek Cells.* Truth be told, at this moment the cheek cell POA test is still a bit ahead of the cutting edge. POA (aka palmitoleic acid) is a long-chain fatty acid that is produced by your body when you turn carbohydrate into fat. The proportion of POA in fat cells of heavy people is higher than in thin people[74]. More importantly, when both thin and heavy people are fed more carbohydrate and less fat, blood and fat cell contents of POA go up[75-77]. Thus POA is a biomarker for that point when your body can't immediately burn or store as glycogen all of the carbohydrates you are eating. Simply put, when your body increases its production of POA, this means that you are eating too much carbohydrate (and perhaps protein).

Okay, so why test POA in cheek cells? First, cheek cells can be collected by rubbing the inside of your cheek with a cotton swab (i.e., not having to bite your lip and prick your finger for blood). Second, cheek cells 'turn over' (i.e., replacing themselves with newly made cells) every few days, so your cheek cell fatty acids reflect your last week's metabolism. Taken together, these two factors indicate that cheek cells are easy to collect and give a prompt indication of your body's metabolic tolerance of your recent diet.

What we currently know about POA is that it goes down when people go on a low carbohydrate diet and it goes up when they eat lots of carbs. But perhaps more importantly, as dietary carbohydrates are increased, some people develop much higher POA levels than others. This suggests that people vary a lot one from another in their responses to increased dietary carbs – some of us are more tolerant of carbohydrate, and some of us less so. Thus the POA levels in your cheek cells appear to be a very sensitive indicator of your personal carbohydrate tolerance.

At the time of this writing, we are testing how accurately cheek cells reflect blood POA levels, and we are also determining if blood POA levels predict who is likely to gain weight if they increase their dietary carbohydrates. We would love to tell you that managing your cheek cell POA content by adjusting your dietary carbs will guide you to the specific diet that will keep you lean. Truthfully, we are not quite there yet. But within a year, we will be.

*HUFA (EPA, DHA, AA) Testing From Cheek Cells.* In Chapter 8, we told you about your need for omega-3 fats, and suggested that you might get a blood test to check your omega-3 levels. As with the POA test, there is the potential that your omega-3 test could also be done using cheek cells. But as with the cheek cell POA test, we are not quite there yet.

The other important fatty acid in cell membranes is arachidonic acid (AA). This omega-6 HUFA is tightly (and positively) linked with insulin sensitivity; and because it is the dominant fatty acid in the membranes of human muscle cells, it is also the target for oxygen free radicals (aka reactive oxygen species, or ROS). We have early research results linking prolonged exercise to HUFA damage from ROS, and this in turn suggests that cheek cell AA might be a valid measure of exercise-induced membrane damage. Again, this is a bit in front of the cutting edge, but the odds are that this might be a useful test for oxidative stress and over-training.

## Summary

The goal of personalized nutrition is to give you accurate information to guide you on your quest for better performance and well-being. As noted above, some of this is a work in progress, but the two current tools we strongly recommend are measuring your blood ketones with a self-administered blood test and determining your body composition (either once or preferably twice) by DXA testing. In addition, if you don't eat much fish or take fish oil supplements, you should consider obtaining an omega-3 blood test (www.omega3test.com). As for the POA and omega-3 tests on cheek cells and breath ketones, we hope to see progress on these within a year, and will post updates on our website (www.artandscienceoflowcarb.com) when new information is available.

# Chapter 11
# SAMPLE MENUS AND RECIPES

*Eating The Right Stuff*

There are many resources to help you get started on a low carbohydrate diet. Not all of the low carbohydrate diet books and cookbooks are 100% in line with our operational definition of a 'well formulated low carbohydrate diet'. If you have low carb cookbooks and recipes you may need to tweak them to ensure the carb count is low enough, protein is moderate, and the right types of fat are emphasized.

When trying to determine what you actually eat on a daily basis, keep these seven important principles in mind.

1. Low in Carbs
   - Enough to induce nutritional ketosis and accelerate fat burning
   - Less than 50 g/day for most people

2. Moderate Protein
   - 0.6 to 1.0 grams per pound of lean body mass

3. Enough Fat
   - Majority of energy
   - Variable depending on goals of weight loss or maintenance

4.  The Right Kinds of Fat
    - Eat monos and saturates for fuel
    - Limit high polyunsaturated sources (soy, corn, cottonseed)

5.  Mineral Management
    - Supplement sodium 2 g/day
    - Replace magnesium to stop muscle cramps

6.  When in Doubt, Eat Less Carbs

7.  When in Doubt, Eat More Fat

## The Right Stuff

To help you get started, you need to stock your refrigerator/freezer and pantry with the right stuff. Here's a list of common items we have in our kitchen.

Avocado
Bacon
Broth
Butter (consider buying Irish butter)
Cheese (hard)
Cream (heavy or whipping)
Eggs
Fish (salmon, tuna, sardines, and herring)
Fruits (berries, olives, tomatoes, lemons, limes)
Mayonnaise (made with olive or canola oil, not soybean oil)
Meats (beef, chicken, pork)
Nuts and seeds
Oils (olive, canola, coconut, high oleic safflower)
Pork rinds
Salami
Salmon

Sausage

Sour cream

Splenda – liquid (www.sweetzfree.com)

Vegetables

Xylitol (available at www.globalsweet.com)

Yogurt (Greek, whole milk)

## Meal Ideas

To spark some creativity, here are ideas for breakfast, lunch and dinner meals.

### Breakfast Options

#### Scrambled eggs with sides of spinach and sausage

Scrambled eggs…2-3 large + 1 Tbsp butter

Shredded mozzarella cheese…1 oz

Pork sausage…2 links

Chopped frozen spinach, boiled…3/4 cup + 1.5 Tbsp butter

#### Cheese omelet and Canadian bacon

Scrambled eggs…2 large + ¼ cup egg beaters + 1.5 Tbsp butter

Shredded cheddar cheese…1 oz

Grilled Canadian bacon…2 oz

#### Ham and asparagus with cauliflower hash browns

Ham slices wrapped around grilled buttered asparagus…4 oz ham +

Asparagus…8 stalks + 1.5 Tbsp butter

Cauliflower hash browns…1/2 cup + 2 Tbsp butter

## Fried eggs with cauliflower hash browns

Fried eggs...2 large

Cauliflower, chopped 3/4 C

Green pepper chopped...1/4 C

Butter... ½ Tbsp

Olive oil...1 Tbsp

Bacon...2 slices

## Eggs Benedict with cauliflower/cheddar patties

Poached eggs...2 large

Hollandaise sauce...1/4 cup (recipe below)

Canadian bacon...2 slices

Cauliflower, chopped...1/2 cup

Olive oil..1 Tbsp + butter...2 Tbsp

Cheddar cheese, shredded...1/4 cup

Egg substitute, liquid...1/8 cup

(Alternatives: serve eggs Benedict over a bed of lightly steamed spinach [Florentine variation] or over sliced avocado [huevos Benedict])

## Cheese omelet with ham and salsa

Eggs, scrambled...2 large

Cream, half and half...2 Tbsp

Swiss cheese...0.5 oz

Cream cheese...1 1/2 Tbsp

Ham, chopped...1 oz

Olive oil...1/2 Tbls + butter...2 Tbsp

Salsa...1/4 cup

### Fried eggs with mushrooms and sausage

Fried eggs... 2 large + 1 Tbsp butter

Sautéed mushrooms... ½ cup + 1 Tbsp butter

Sausage link...2

## Lunch Options

### Broiled salmon and a side salad

Broiled Atlantic salmon...4 oz + 1 Tbsp butter

Side salad: mixed baby greens...2 1/2 cups

Diced tomatoes...1/4 cup

Chopped onion...1/8 cup

Feta cheese...1 oz

Black and green olives...4 each

Blue cheese dressing...1 1/2 Tbsp

### Cheeseburger with sautéed mushrooms and peppers

Hamburger (70% lean/30% fat)...3 oz

American cheese...1 oz

Iceberg lettuce...1/2 cup

Red tomato...2 slices

Red onions...3 slices

Sautéed sweet bell peppers...1/4 cup +
mushrooms...1/4 cup + 2 Tbsp olive oil

## Greek salad

>   Roasted chicken breast…5 oz + 1.5 Tbsp olive oil
>
>   4 Calamata olives
>
>   Shredded romaine lettuce…2 cups
>
>   Tomato slices
>
>   Red onions, sliced…1/4 cup
>
>   Feta cheese….1.5 oz
>
>   Balsamic vinegar…1 Tbsp
>
>   Olive oil…1 Tbsp

## Tuna salad on bed of tomato and cucumber slices

>   Tuna, canned in oil….3.25 oz
>
>   Celery…2 stalks diced
>
>   Mayo (made with canola oil)…2 Tbsp
>
>   Almonds, slivered
>
>   Tomato…3 slices
>
>   Cucumber sliced….1/4 cup

## Turkey/Cheese/pickle roll ups

>   Swiss cheese…2 oz
>
>   Turkey deli sliced…3 oz
>
>   Ham deli sliced…2 slices
>
>   Mayo (made with canola oil)…2 Tbsp
>
>   Dill pickle….4 slices
>
>   Celery…2 stalks
>
>   Cream cheese…1 1/2 Tbsp

### Caesar salad with steak

Lettuce, romaine, shredded...1 1/2 cup

Cucumber, sliced...1/4 cup + tomatoes, red, diced...1/4 cup

Mushrooms, sliced

Beef loin tri tip (broiled)...2.5 oz

Caesar salad dressing...2 Tbsp

Parmesan cheese, grated...2 Tbsp

### Grilled chicken salad

Romaine lettuce... 3 1/2 cups

Chicken breast (with skin)... 3 oz

Avocado... ½ item

Blue cheese dressing...4 Tbsp

## Dinner Options

### Sirloin with sautéed mushrooms and cauliflower mashed potatoes

Beef sirloin tips...3 oz

Olive oil...1 1/2 Tbsp

Sautéed mushrooms...1/4 cup

Olive oil cooking spray

Cauliflower "mashed potatoes": boiled cauliflower...1 cup +

shredded cheddar cheese...1 oz

Butter...1 Tbsp

Sugar free jello...1/2 cup

## Pork chops and cauliflower "mashed potatoes"

> Pork chops…3 oz
>
> String beans…1/2 cup, boiled + 1 1/2 Tbsp olive oil
>
> Cauliflower…1/2 cup, mashed + 1.5 Tbsp butter
>
> Shredded cheddar cheese…1/4 cup

## Taco-less tacos

> Ground beef crumbles (70% fat/30% lean)….3 oz + 1 Tbsp olive oil
>
> Sour cream…2 Tbsp
>
> Diced red tomatoes…1/4 cup
>
> 6 black olives
>
> Chopped chives…2 tsp
>
> Avocado…½
>
> Leaf iceberg lettuce…1 1/2 cup

## Buffalo style chicken salad with creamy blueberry dessert

> Roast chicken breast…4 oz
>
> Hot sauce….1 tsp + butter…2 Tbsp
>
> Blue cheese dressing…1 1/2 Tbsp
>
> Romaine lettuce…shredded 1 1/2 cup
>
> Tomato…2 slices
>
> Almonds, slivered…1/8 cup
>
> Dessert: cream cheese…1/3 cup, heavy cream… 3 Tbsp, lemon juice…1 tsp, frozen blueberries unsweetened…1/4 cup

## Chicken/Swiss roll ups w/ sautéed spinach & cauliflower pilaf

Chicken breast, pounded thin…3 oz

Swiss cheese, sliced…1 oz

Spinach, chopped, boiled…1/4 cup

Olive oil…1 Tbsp + butter…2 Tbsp

+ lemon zest 1/2 Tbsp + garlic…1/2 clove

Parmesan cheese, grated…1/2 oz

Cauliflower, chopped…1/2 cup

Olive oil…1/2 Tbsp + Butter…2 Tbsp

## Roast beef w/ horseradish cream sauce

Top round beef…3.5 oz

Green beans…½ cup + 1 Tbsp butter

Mozzarella cheese…1 1/2 oz

Red tomato…1 item

Basil…1 tsp

Butter…2 Tbsp

Horseradish sauce: prepared horseradish…
1 Tbsp + mayonnaise…1 Tbsp

## High Fat Recipes

If you are struggling with ways to specifically increase fat, then try these recipes reprinted from "The Art and Science of Low Carbohydrate Living". You can also download a 7 day diet plan:

http://www.artandscienceoflowcarb.com/wp-content/
uploads/2011/06/7-Day-Menus.pdf

## Sautéed kale with garlic and olive oil

Ingredients:

- 20 or so kale leaves 6" to 10" long (1-2 bunches in the market)
- 2 cloves of garlic peeled and chopped (about 2 teaspoons)
- 3 tablespoons olive oil
- ¼ teaspoon salt

Rinse the kale in cold water and strip the flesh from the stems, discard the stems and tear the flesh into postage stamp-sized pieces, allow to drain in a colander or sieve.

Brown the garlic lightly in the olive oil over medium heat in a large skillet, then add the shredded kale and salt to the hot oil and cover. Reduce the heat to simmer covered for ten minutes, stirring once or twice so it cooks evenly. Serves 3-4, 10 grams of fat per serving.

Alternative: rather than olive oil, use an ounce or two of finely chopped sow belly, fried lightly before adding the garlic. This dish can be made with collards as well.

## Cucumber yogurt salad

Ingredients:

- 6 medium or 4 large cucumbers peeled and sliced
- 4 sprigs of dill, chopped (about 2 teaspoons)
- 2 cups full fat plain yogurt (**not** the sweetened vanilla flavor)
- 2 tablespoons fresh lemon juice
- 2 cloves of garlic, peeled
- 4 tablespoons olive oil, preferably extra virgin
- ½ teaspoon salt
- ¼ teaspoon finely ground black pepper

Put the dill, garlic, olive oil, lemon juice, pepper, and salt in an 8-12 cup food processor and blend with the metal blade until smooth. Add the yogurt and blend briefly until well mixed.

Pour the yogurt mix over the cucumbers in a covered bowl and chill.

Makes 4-6 servings, each containing 12 grams of fat and 4 grams of carbohydrate.

For a nice presentation, serve in small bowls with 5-6 Belgium endive leaves as scoops.

## Creamed spinach

Ingredients:

- 2 pounds fresh spinach
- 2 medium onions finely chopped
- 2-3 cloves of garlic finely chopped
- 1 cup heavy cream
- 2 tablespoons butter
- 2 tablespoons olive oil
- Salt and pepper
- Parmesan cheese (optional)

Wash and drain spinach and remove tough stems. In a large pot, sauté onions and garlic in butter and olive oil until translucent. Add spinach, constantly stir and press down until leaves are wilted. Add cream and cook until desired texture. Add salt and pepper to taste. Top with shaved parmesan cheese (optional).

**French Fried Green Beans**

Finger food to go with a steak or burger, or just by themselves for the fun of it!

Ingredients:

- 1 pound of fresh green beans
- 1 teaspoon coarse sea salt
- ½ teaspoon black peppercorns or rose peppercorns
- ¼ teaspoon garlic powder
- ½ teaspoon dried Italian seasoning mix
- 1 egg white

Pre-heat a deep fat fryer to 240°F (hot) –preferably filled with high oleic safflower oil

Rinse green beans, trim, and pat dry on a towel

Grind spices together in a mortar and pestle

Whip egg white until foamy, then coat the green beans in egg,

Put egg-coated beans in a 1-qt plastic bag and dust with ground spices, shake vigorously, and drop into hot oil. Fry for 2-3 minutes. Remove when the egg coating just starts to brown.

**Tomato bisque**

This recipe is best if you have ripe tomatoes and fresh basil from your garden, otherwise use plum (roma) tomatoes from the store.

Ingredients:

- 1 large onion sliced ¼ inch thick
- 6 large or 12 small tomatoes (the total volume should be 2-3 cups)

- 10-15 fresh basil leaves

- ¼ cup light olive oil

- ½ teaspoon finely ground black pepper

- 4 cups home-made chicken broth

- 1 cup medium (25% fat) or heavy (40% fat) cream

Rinse the tomatoes and basil leaves in cold water and drain on a towel.

Put olive oil and onions in a medium (3-4 quart) pot and brown over medium heat for about 5 minutes. The onions should end up light brown, soft, and translucent.

Cut the tomatoes in half and add them along with the basil leaves and pepper. Cover and simmer for 10 minutes, until the tomatoes are soft and cooked through.

Allow to cool for 5 minutes and place tomato/onion mixture in a food processor and blend for 60 seconds, pulsing frequently to be sure all large hunks are chopped fine.

Rinse the cooking pot, place a large sieve over it, and strain the blended tomato onion mix through it, discarding any solids that don't go thru the sieve. Depending on how smooth you want the texture of the soup, you can choose the sieve mesh size from coarse to fine.

Add the chicken broth to the tomato onion puree and warm over low heat. Heat until it just starts to steam (160-170 °F) -- don't let it boil!

Take soup off the heat and whisk in the heavy cream.

Salt to taste (the amount depends if your chicken broth was salted).

Serve warm. Serves 6. Provides 20-25 grams fat and 5 grams carbohydrate per 10 oz serving,

## Wedgie

Ingredients:

- 1 head of iceberg lettuce, stripped of wilted outer leaves, rinsed and drained
- ½ cup of crumbled blue cheese
- ½ cup of bacon fried lightly crisp and chopped
- 1 cup of sliced or diced fresh tomatoes
- 1 cup of sliced or diced cucumber
- 1 cup of yogurt blue cheese dressing (recipe below).

Slice the lettuce into quarters through the stem and remove the core from each piece.

Slice each quarter again to make equal wedges (eights) and lay the two narrow edges together in the center of a salad plate.

Arrange the toppings in the 'central valley' – for example put cucumber and tomatoes on either end and the blue cheese and bacon in the middle.

Drizzle 4 oz of the yogurt blue cheese dressing over the top when served.

Serves 4.   Fat content 30 grams per serving.


## Breakfast Berry Smoothie

Ingredients:

- 3 oz fresh or frozen (unsweetened) berries (strawberries, blue-berries, or raspberries)
- ¼ cup whipping (or heavy) cream
- 1 tablespoon light olive oil
- 2 tablespoons unflavored whey protein powder (delactosed)

- sweetener of choice (e.g., 1 tablespoon xylitol and 1 packet Splenda)
- 2-3 oz ice

Blend the ingredients at high speed until smooth (30-60 seconds)

Protein 15 grams, Fat 25-30 grams, Carbs 10 grams, Calories 330-380

## Breakfast Mocca Smoothie

Ingredients:

- 4 oz coffee ice (frozen in ice cube tray – if frozen as a big lump in a cup or bowel, it's hard to blend)
- ¼ cup whipping or heavy cream
- 1 tablespoon unsweetened cocoa powder
- 1 tablespoon light olive oil
- 2 tablespoons unflavored whey protein powder (delactosed)
- sweetener of choice (e.g., 1 tablespoon xylitol and 1 packet Splenda)

Blend the ingredients at high speed until smooth (30-60 seconds)

Protein 15 grams, Fat 25-30 grams, Carbs 6 grams, Calories 310-350

## Blender Hollandaise Sauce

This is a quick (3 minute prep time) and delicious alternative to the traditional hollandaise whisked together over a double boiler.

Ingredients:

- 4 oz butter (one stick)
- 3 egg yolks
- 2 tablespoons fresh lemon juice
- Pinch of paprika

Heat the butter in a small pan until it just starts to sizzle (but don't brown)

Put the egg yolks, lemon juice and paprika to a blender and pulse briefly to mix.

With the blender running, slowly pour the hot butter into the blender (10-15 seconds).

Pulse briefly until color is uniform and serve warm.

Serves 4. Use over steamed vegetables and for eggs Benedict.

Protein 2 grams, Fat 26 grams, Carbs 1 gram, Calories 246

## Yogurt blue cheese dressing

Commercial blue cheese dressings abound out there, so why should I make my own?

Answer: Better taste, better nutrition, and the right kind of fat. And if you need another reason, this recipe can be made in quantity and stored in your freezer in single serving doses. Spend 15 minutes making a batch now, and get 10 servings whenever you want them later.

Ingredients:

- 2 cloves of garlic,

- 10 fresh basil leaves

- 2 tablespoons fresh lemon juice

- ¼ cup olive oil

- 4 cups plain unsweetened yogurt (full or low fat, not fat-free and definitely **not** vanilla!)

- 8 oz crumbled blue cheese

- 1/8 teaspoon finely ground black pepper

- 1 teaspoon salt

Put the garlic, basil, lemon juice, olive oil, pepper, salt, and 4 oz (half) of the blue cheese in a blender or food processor and process until smooth. Add the yogurt and pulse until well mixed. Add the other 4 oz of blue cheese and process briefly to mix (but not blend).

Parcel out ½ cup units into snack zip-lock bags, squeezing out any extra air. Put in a container and freeze.

When needed, take individual ½ cup units out of the freezer and thaw for a few minutes in cool water.

Makes 10 half-cup servings, each containing 16 grams of fat.

## Honey basil dressing

Ingredients:

- 10 cloves of roasted garlic
- 20 fresh medium or 10 large basil leaves
- ¼ cup unsweetened rice vinegar (find it in the Asian foods section of your grocery)
- ¼ cup honey
- 2 packets of Splenda or 2 level tablespoons xylitol
- 1 cup light (not extra virgin) olive oil
- ½ teaspoon salt

The best way to roast garlic is to get a covered ceramic garlic roaster, slice the tops off a full garlic bulb, drizzle it with a tablespoon of olive oil and roast in the over for 45 min at 400 °F. Alternatively use a metal muffin tin, place the trimmed garlic bulb base down, drizzle with olive oil, cover each bulb with aluminum foil, and bake for 30-40 min at 400 °F. When done, the garlic cloves are soft and starting to push up out of the holes you cut in the top of each clove.

Put the roasted garlic cloves, basil leaves, rice vinegar and honey into a food processor or blender and process until very smooth (at least 2 minutes). Add the olive oil, sweetener, and salt. Blend until well mixed. Refrigerate extra in a closed container.

Makes 12 one oz servings, each containing 20 grams of fat and 5 grams of carbohydrate.

## Sun-dried tomato caper dip (tapenade)

Here's a simple way to dry tomatoes. Using a sharp knife, slice ripe tomatoes in ¼ inch thick slices blot dry on a paper towel, and lay on waxed paper in a dish in the bottom of the microwave. If you have a microwave shelf, cover it with more tomato slices as well. Run the microwave for 5 minutes at 30% power (defrost) and then for 60 minutes at 10% power. A 1000 Watt microwave puts out 100 Watts at 10% power, so it's making about as much heat as a 100 Watt light bulb, and the tomato slices should be slightly warm but not hot. Check the tomatoes after each hour, turning and rearranging as needed to help them dry evenly, repeating the same 5/60 minute heating cycle each time. This will dry 3-4 pounds of tomatoes in about 5 hrs. When done, they should be leathery in texture and still dark red. Do not dry them to black crispy wisps.

Ingredients:

- 3 oz of dried tomatoes (from 1.5 to 2 pounds of fresh tomatoes)
- 2 oz non-pareil pickled capers, lightly rinsed and drained
- 20 fresh basil leaves
- 3-5 cloves roasted garlic
- 1 packet Splenda or one level tablespoon xylitol
- 2 tablespoons unsweetened rice vinegar or wine vinegar
- 1 cup light olive oil

Add everything together in a food processor and blend until the tomato and basil are down to fine bits. The flavor is best if made at least an hour before serving. Remaining dip can be refrigerated for a week.

Each tablespoon contains 10 grams of fat.

## Maple walnut ice cream

Ingredients:

- ½ cup English walnuts
- 2 tablespoons butter
- 2 tablespoons real maple syrup
- 4 cups heavy or whipping cream
- 2/3 cup xylitol
- 8 packets Splenda
- 2-3 drops of artificial maple flavor

Chop the walnuts to pea size. Put the nuts in a small frying pan with the butter and heat over low heat until the nuts just start to brown. Add the maple syrup to nuts and butter and stir gently over low heat until the syrup thickens and coats the nuts. Take off the heat and allow to cool. When cool, the nuts should harden into firm sticky lumps.

Mix the cream and sweeteners together and stir with a spoon until all are dissolved. Add the maple flavor and put in an ice cream maker, churning until it is thick enough to form a stable mound on a spoon. Break apart the lumps of sugary nuts and drop them into the ice cream and churn only until well distributed. Put in the freezer to firm up.

Makes 10 half-cup servings, each containing 25-40 grams of fat and 4 grams of carbs.

## Chocolate pecan ice cream

Although slightly more work than the maple walnut ice cream, this decadent "French-style" custard-based ice cream made with egg yolks and heavy cream delivers an even richer and silkier texture.

Ingredients:

- 4 cups heavy or whipping cream
- 9 large egg yolks
- ½ cup xylitol
- 3 tablespoons unsweetened cocoa powder
- 1 teaspoon vanilla extract
- 8 packets Splenda or 3-4 drops liquid Splenda
- 3 tablespoons butter
- ¾ cup chopped pecans
- 3 tablespoons vanilla sugar-free syrup (e.g., Da Vinci)

In a saucepan, warm 3½ cups of the cream on medium heat until bubbles form around the edges.

Combine the egg yolks, remaining ½ cup cream, xylitol, and cocoa in a metal bowl. Whisk until the mixture is smooth. Pour about ½ cup of the warm cream into the egg mixture, whisking constantly until smooth and the xylitol begins to dissolve.

Pour the egg mixture back into the saucepan containing warm cream. Cook over medium heat stirring constantly until custard thickens (don't boil). The custard should leave a clear trail when a finger is drawn through it. Stir in vanilla and Splenda.

Place entire mixture into a bowl and cool. You can cool the bowl faster by placing it in a larger bowl filled with ice cubes and water. Stir frequently until mixture cools to room temperature. Then chill in freezer for an hour before churning.

Chop the pecans to pea size. In a frying pan melt the butter and add the pecans. Cook over medium heat for a couple minutes stirring constantly to cover the pecans with butter until they are brown. Add the sugar-free syrup and continue to stir constantly until the syrup thickens and coats the pecans. Take off the heat, allow to cool, and place in the freezer. The nuts should harden into firm sticky lumps.

Take chilled custard out of the freezer and pour into an ice cream maker. Churn until volume expands and thickens. Break apart the candied pecans and stir into the ice cream mixture until well distributed. Put into containers and store in freezer.

## Blueberry cheesecake

Ingredients:

- 2 packets plain unsweetened gelatin
- 1 cup xylitol  (alternative ½ cup xylitol and 6 packets Splenda).
- 1 ½ cups water
- 12 oz creamed cheese
- 1/4 cup light olive oil
- 2 teaspoons vanilla extract
- 2 cups fresh blueberries (or sliced strawberries)

Heat the water to boiling, remove from heat and sprinkle the gelatin powder in while stirring vigorously until it is dissolved (clear).

Put the creamed cheese, olive oil, xylitol, and vanilla in a food processor, pour in the hot gelatin solution, and process until smooth.

Rinse the blueberries, pat dry, and put in the bottom of a 9-inch pie plate. Pour the still warm gelatin-cheese mix over the berries and chill in the refrigerator until it sets (30-60 min).

Makes 12 4-5 oz servings, each with 15 grams of fat and 4 grams of carbohydrate.

Alternatively, distribute the berries into 6 'snack size' Zip-Loc' bags and pour in enough cheesecake liquid to fill each bag. Squeeze out any air, seal immediately, and refrigerate). The sealed bags keep for up to a week refrigerated and a day unrefrigerated.

# Chapter 12

# LOW CARB ATHLETES

*Personal Observations From Athletes Pushing The Envelope*

Change is never led by consensus. That's what pioneers are for. The Union Pacific Railroad didn't invent the airplane, and the New York Times didn't invent the Internet. True innovation is usually disruptive of traditional business or societal norms, and thus the consensus response to a new idea – no matter how good – is usually denial.

Given this perspective, it is not surprising that the transformation of sports nutrition by the low carbohydrate message is being led by individual pioneers willing to step (or run) outside the box – not by the mainstream experts. This chapter presents, in their own words, the stories of seven low carb athlete pioneers.

## Tony Ricci, M.S., CSCS, LDN, CISSN, CNS
## High-Performance Coach/Sports Nutritionist

In 27 years of experience in human performance training and nutrition, I have heard of just about every dietary practice ever considered. I have intentionally practiced a multitude of dietary approaches throughout my career from spending a full year as a vegetarian to more transient use of ultra-high protein diets. Through trial and error I have found that my body responds best to a ketogenic diet. While consuming a high carbohydrate (60% of energy) diet consisting of 3100 Calories per day I gained weight watching my body fat climb to 12%. Currently in my 40's on a well designed ketogenic diet as recommended by Jeff and Steve, I consume up to 4200 calories per day while maintaining 6-7% body fat. This transformation has resulted in an increase in my power to mass ratio and allows a high level of performance in a range of activities. Equally, if not more important, is the efficiency with which I operate in every facet of my life. My energy level in a keto-adapted state is constant, and never undulates. My quality of sleep, focus and cognitive abilities are elevated. For me personally one of the most profound effects of eating a very low carbohydrate diet is the satiation. On high carbohydrate diets I was always hungry on an incessant quest for food. My message to all athletes regardless of your sports discipline; you may need 3-4 weeks to fully adapt when training intensely, but once you do, I am confident you will enjoy performance and quality of life benefits.

## Andrea Hudy, Assistant Athletic Director for Sports Performance, University of Kansas

My interest in a low carb diet began as a personal journey but quickly turned professional. Throughout my career I have been exposed to just about every type of nutrition system. Through personal trial and error, I have found that low carb works best for me and some of the athletes I train. I began my low carb nutrition program as a way to help with my personal endurance performance – specifically, training for a half marathon. I was interested in increasing my aerobic capacity and having more energy. I was immediately pleased with the results as it pertains to my aerobic performance and increased energy, but was also pleased to find that it left my appetite satisfied and I soon began dropping weight.

There is a misconception out there that a low carb diet has to be a boring diet, but I find that not to be true. On this nutritional program I am still able to enjoy the foods I love (fruits, nuts, vegetables, etc) which leaves me less likely to stray. I felt great during my training and competition which motivated me to continue low carb. I have since competed in seven half marathons, each time improving. I credit this to low carb.

After my own success on the low carb diet, I was confident in recommending it to my athletes. I had several athletes who were interested in increasing their sports performance while losing weight at the same time. We all know college athletes have a lot of distractions but I was comfortable that, given the convenience and simplicity of the program, this program was something they could stick to. Immediately I received positive feedback. Not only with their training intensity, but an added benefit was that their cramping decreased.

## Low Carb Diets Plus VESPA

A recent discovery by our friend Peter Defty has been the combined use of a low carbohydrate diet with VESPA, a naturally-occurring peptide extracted from the predatory wasp Vespa mandarinia (www.vespapower.com). Given that this species of wasp can travel vast distances on its modest body fat reserves, VESPA was developed as an aide to optimize your access to body fat for fuel during prolonged events. As a coach and former competitive trail runner who manages the diet, training and progress for several high level ultra endurance athletes, Peter has made the empiric observation that VESPA works best when athletes go through a period of keto-adaptation. Using a regimen he has named Optimized Fat Metabolism (OFM), Peter's dietary advice during training is very similar to ours as laid out in 'The Art and Science of Low Carbohydrate Living', although he advises some individuals to add some carbs before and during competition.

To date, the scientific literature (as in prospective randomized trials) on VESPA is scant. It is admittedly difficult to do such research in athletes participating in ultra-endurance events (e.g., 50-100+ mile foot-races lasting 6-30 hr). However numerous athletes report being able to participate in successive races of these lengths with less than 2 weeks recovery, as well as 200-3000 mile bike races lasting 1-14 days. These improbable race tempos indicate that both performance and recovery are markedly improved through a combination of low carbohydrate diet and VESPA. Below are three ultra-endurance runners' stories of low carbohydrate and/or keto-adapted athletes using VESPA.

## Bettie Smith, 60, Cool, CA

I guess for people running ultras, everyone has at least one chronic issue. Mine was my stomach. It's always been cranky, and since I started running ultras in 2007 it had just gotten worse and worse. Finally, after an endoscope exam last year revealed an eroded stomach lining, but no known cause, and spending a couple of races periodically doubled over while it felt like someone was spraying acid on my stomach lining, I knew it time to get completely serious about finding a solution or quit running altogether.

All along I'd been trying various fuels, electrolytes, etc. in training, all without any success but some truly memorable crashes. I'd heard good things about VESPA but since I'm just an average runner I had felt I couldn't really justify using it. A friend gave me a couple of packets to try, probably so I'd just quit talking about trying it and just do it. I noticed a subtle energy difference immediately.

Enter Peter Defty, who told me it was the very carbs I loved that were the source of my intestinal woes. They were keeping me from burning fat and forcing my body to chase my calories to prevent bonking. I give him full credit for his advice about a lower carb diet and electrolyte use, and for his product, VESPA, for solving those issues. When I started with VESPA I hadn't any intention of really changing my diet. But after talking to Peter, I did some reading and made a few adjustments, and then a few more because I was feeling so much better overall! Now I even train without Prilosec.

A month later, my first race using VESPA was the 2011 Way Too Cool where I finally broke 6 hours on a 50K. Then in Silver States 50, I won first in my age group!

I've changed my diet completely now and feel like a new person. I've eliminated wheat and other grains almost entirely, eating more meats and fats than I ever have in my life. I'd never eaten many prepared processed foods before anyway and I've always loved fruit and vegetables, so that was easy to do. I try to love vegetables more than fruit now though.

It's been a little over a year since I started using VESPA and made the dietary changes. I realized recently that I haven't hit a low in a race or training since I did. I ran Cascade Crest 100 Mile Trail Race in September 2011 without a pacer, staying alert and focused the entire time, taking an hour and 10 minutes off my PR and having what was truly a perfect day. And in three weeks I felt like I could do it again.

Training or racing, I can run with very little additional fuel. I have learned to recognize early on how I feel and when I need to add a few carbs to the mix. I can't begin to explain how wonderful it feels; to run knowing I can eat something if I need to and looking forward to it when I do, to run in complete happiness instead of in a fog, to run knowing I can just keep going until I want to stop, because that's what it's all about for me. I now truly enjoy every step of way.

## Doug Berlin, Owner, Gold's Gym: Sterling/Herndon/Ashburn/Reston, VA

Health and fitness are my life. I have been working out since the age of thirteen, have trained in fitness disciplines ranging from body building to my current sport of ultramarathon trail running. As the majority owner of four Gold's Gyms in suburban Washington D.C. I spend my 11+ hour work day on my feet training/coaching athletes, signing new clients, working with my managers and even policing the locker room...it never stops. Each weekday I lift weights for 45 minutes and run 8-10 miles. Saturday morning I am out the door early for a 30 mile run.

In early 2011, I decided to try a product called VESPA which had begun to get a small but strong following in the ultramarathon scene. I immediately noticed I was not chasing my calories anymore on long runs and races and recovering much faster. After 4 months I contacted VESPA and spoke with Peter Defty about the product. I was curious to know more because it was inconceivable I was performing so well on so little. Peter started telling me that if I wanted to improve my performance to another level I needed to Optimize Fat Metabolism (OFM) by sharply reducing my carbohydrate consumption on a daily basis, increasing my consumption of fat to where it constituted 50-60% of my calories and maintain a moderate level of protein from fresh animal sources. Then, prior to a race, he said I could "sneak" some carbs into my diet and use them as needed during a race. Naturally this went against everything I have ever heard about nutrition for athletes. To prove there was sound science behind what he was saying, Peter sent me a book list and a copy of "The Art & Science of Low Carbohydrate Living".

Making the dietary shift has been monumental! The difference is night-and-day from the energy swings I was having on my old diet. Now, I have the boundless energy of an eighteen year old. What is more amazing is the more fat I incorporated into my diet, the leaner I got. In the past year, at age 45, I have gone from 7% body fat to 5.3% body fat. I am 6' 6" and weigh 200 pounds. When I shifted the diet, my weight did not change, just body composition. Naturally my performance skyrocketed and I set a string of PRs at various races in late 2011 including 100 mile runs. What is really amazing is the recovery. It's insane!

## John Rutherford

I raced bicycles competitively for 6 seasons, from the age of 13-19. After 2 years of racing - and placing 3rd at the U.S. Jr. National Championships in the 20 kilometer time trial, I was invited to attend National Team selection camp. On the final day of the 2 week camp, I was indeed invited to join the team, but advised that I needed to lose at least 10 pounds off of my then 160 lb frame.

My solution was to further restrict fat, increase volume, and restrict calories. Ultimately this proved effective, but my energy levels were subject to massive swings. The diet was sustainable during the racing season (through discipline) but thoroughly unenjoyable in both substance and effect. Each September I would promptly regain the 10-15 pounds of adipose fat that I had shed through volume and calorie restriction during the previous winter's base phase. I routinely found that on certain completely random days,

I would have very little energy or motivation to train, and each race became a battle against the inevitable bonk. I maintained my competitive edge at shorter distances (less than an hour), but consistently suffered with fueling during longer and multi-day events. This, and other factors, led to emotional and physical burnout half-way through my second season as a full-time, semi-professional cyclist. I hung up the bike and resumed life as a "normal" person. Freed from the strictures of a coach counting calories for me, my diet shifted back to something more classically American. I still wasn't eating fast food or drinking regular soda, but I wasn't weighing my food or blotting the grease off my pizza either.

I joined the Marine Corps after 3 relatively sedentary years in college. The military turned me into a runner, and after 2 years dedicated to intense flight training, I got the itch to compete again. Cycling wasn't practical, and truth be told I still had a fairly bad taste in my mouth. I'd lost love for that sport in particular, but not for the lifestyle and challenge of reaching peak physical form. Somewhere along the way I got it in my head to someday run a 100 mile ultra-marathon. This idea was planted by a high-school chemistry teacher who would wear his Western States Endurance Run belt buckle (awarded for completing that race in under 24 hours; "One Hundred Miles, One Day"). I was intrigued by the challenge of the distance, not least because of the trouble I'd had with longer events in the past.

That first year, 2004, I began training in June with the initial goal of a trail marathon in November. It was something of a death march toward the end, but I was nevertheless inspired by attaining this early goal. The following January brought my first road marathon. I finished in 3:17, tantalizingly close to the Boston Marathon qualifying time for my age group: 3:10. I followed this effort with my first 50 miler at American River in early April 2005. Countless 50k and marathon distance races followed over the next two years, including a 2:51:20 marathon PR at Boston. Throughout, I continued to live, train, and fuel on a high carbohydrate diet. Predictably, my original problem persisted.

I attempted my first 100 miler in the summer of 2006 at Tahoe Rim Trail. While altitude and the preceding month spent training on a treadmill aboard a U.S. Navy aircraft carrier certainly didn't help matters, my fueling was the ultimate cause of my withdrawal at mile 50. Dinner the night before was pasta, breakfast was pancakes, and every 45 minutes of running brought another energy gel. By mile 35, I was both shuffling and hallucinating through the Sierra high country. I had experienced lesser bonks at the 50 mile distance in the recent past, most likely due to the advantages of sea level, but this was different. Discouraged, TRT was my last race before leaving the United States for nearly 2 years deployed overseas.

I returned from my second successive deployment in August of 2008 registered and ready for October's Chicago Marathon. Despite having prepared much as I had in the past, it proved a difficult day with a hard bonk at mile 20. Curiously, I left Chicago more inspired than ever to conquer the 100 mile distance. That winter I signed up for the Vermont 100, to be held in July 2009, and a string of lesser distances throughout the spring. Knowing that the bonk was inevitable, I decided to focus on my in-race fueling. This worked to an extent. I finished Vermont in a respectable 21:42, but not without two debilitating bonks at miles 35 and 62 and a painful multi-week recovery process.

I was hooked on 100s, but realized that I had to fix my fueling problems. I had to try something radically different. Stuck in my mind was the experience of eating the single most delicious thing I have ever had: a butter soaked grilled cheese sandwich in an aid station at mile 88 of the Vermont. My body demanded fat, and counter to my intuition at the time, performed accordingly when I met that need. My last 10 miles were a breeze.

Enter VESPA and OFM. I found through research that there was a small but vocal cohort of trail runners who swore by their high fat, low sugar diets. The following season I decided to experiment, but didn't fully buy into the concept until two days after the Angeles Crest 100. My recovery was exponentially easier and faster than after Vermont one year earlier. Despite running for 6 additional hours over a much more challenging course at altitude (27:45; hydration proved my foe that weekend), my body snapped back very, very quickly.

Completely converted, I ran 50k and 50m PRs the following spring on 250 and 400 in-race Calories, respectively. In June I finished the Western States 100 in 19:30 on something less than 2000 Calories. Ten days later I ran the fastest 8 miles of my life on a 90 degree Washington DC afternoon. My diet during training had transitioned to a focus on unprocessed, high quality saturated and mono-unsaturated fats: cream, butter, extra virgin coconut oil, macadamia butter, salmon, sardines, anchovies, avocados, eggs, raw nuts, chia seeds... Protein and carbohydrate continued to play a role, not least in adding additional palatability, but my emphasis in every meal became fat as the dominant macronutrient. I have maintained roughly the same body weight since experiencing an initial reduction of about 5 pounds, but as I've become more disciplined with OFM I've traded fat for lean muscle. Today, in the off-season waiting to begin the ramp-up for my fourth 100, I find myself consistently sated, high energy, and leaner than ever despite a relatively low training volume.

OFM has completely changed my running. I simply do not suffer now like I did on a high-carbohydrate diet. Ingesting fewer calories over the course of a long run has removed my single most cumbersome barrier to higher performance. Running isn't just easier on OFM, it's more fun, too.

**And finally, two more detailed stories of low carbohydrate athletes:**

### Jay Wortman MD and Isabelle – The Need For Speed

I was always addicted to speed. I bought my first Porsche when I was 17 years old. It was a rusty old 1959 356A but I loved that car and drove it like I was racing on the European rally circuit. Three years later I bought my first motorcycle, a used Kawasaki 650, that I rebuilt in a mechanic friend's basement over the winter. I rode it for only six weeks before t-boning a car and waking up in the hospital with some broken teeth and soft tissue injuries but, otherwise, not seriously injured. I used the insurance settlement to buy a bigger, faster Ducati 750 GT and a Porsche 911. And I took up hang-gliding while still wearing a neck brace from the bike crash.

It was at that time, when I was in my twenties, that I also developed a love for downhill skiing. The sensation of free-fall as I raced down the slopes of various Rocky Mountain ski areas was exhilarating. I combined skiing with hang-gliding and toured the mountain resorts where gliders were allowed on the ski-lifts. Launching a glider while on skis was less gut wrenching than hurling myself off a cliff but it wasn't without its hazards mainly due to the temptation to fly in less than ideal wind conditions.

Eventually, I started to grow up and act more responsibly. I let the hang-glider go after too many of my friends were killed in crashes. The Porsches went mainly because of their cost and the impracticality of air-cooled engines in northern winters. My last Ducati was sold shortly after my son was born.

I look back on those speed-drenched days and marvel at the fact that I actually survived. My life now is very sedate in comparison, with one exception. Okay, maybe two. I still struggle to keep my little diesel Jetta wagon within the posted speed limit. I'll get to that other exception in a minute.

During my youth, I was always thin as a rake. It never occurred to me to exercise. I was active all the time. Whether navigating a D10 bulldozer or riding a big café racer motorcycle, it took strength and effort. Hauling a hang-glider up a mountain was a work-out. I ate like a horse and stayed slim as a rail. During this time I worked in heavy oil-field construction in a physically active job. There was no need to go to the gym. The concepts of diet and exercise never entered my head.

Then, everything changed. I went back to school. Going to med school and, eventually, starting a family were big factors in bringing me back to earth and slowing me down. Ironically, those changes were also contributing factors to the eventual deterioration in my physical health. I started to gain weight not long after starting university. At first it was subtle, I moved up a waist size or two. No big deal. Then, as the years went by and the course loads and stress levels became heavier as I progressed through med school my physical condition deteriorated. I gained more weight and went up some more inches in waist size. It was then that I discovered the benefits of exercising in a gym. I began to do a short but fairly intense workout every morning in the basement gym in the med school. I toned up and my waist size shrank a bit. I also noticed that it helped in other ways, my ability to concentrate improved and there were gains in my academic performance, as well. I still gave no thought to diet.

As med school progressed to residency and the chaotic lifestyle of hospital work and overnight call, I fell off the exercise schedule and my physical condition worsened. Again, I still gave little thought to diet except for the influence of one of my surgical preceptors who was convinced that meat was the cause of all the bowel cancer he was seeing. I stopped eating meat and became a pesco-vegetarian. Equipped with only the scant nutritional instruction typical of a medical education, it also seemed like a good idea to cut down on fats, too. This was the diet I would follow for the next several years, right up to the point where I developed type 2 diabetes at the age of 52.

By this time, my waist had expanded from the 28 inches of those long ago construction days to the more portly 36 inches of my middle aged family life. I was still active, though. I loved golf and played every weekend. I usually walked the course, which is great exercise. The golf did dwindle away after my son was born but in the evenings and on weekends I rode a bicycle to pull the little trailer in which he would ride. And I was still indulging my need for speed with downhill skiing.

I went skiing at Whistler every chance I got. This was the only risky speed related activity that had survived my transition from reckless youth to sedate adulthood. I skied as fast as I could. I recall doing run after run and telling myself each time that I had to slow down or a calamity would surely ensue. There were times that I actually frightened myself with the speed. I was addicted, however, and I just couldn't stop myself. My solution for this dilemma was to take up snowboarding.

By this time, my chances of surviving this high-risk lifestyle of speed addiction had greatly improved. For example, after the death of Sonny Bono in a skiing accident at Lake Tahoe in 1998, I did start wearing a helmet. My health, however, was in decline. Even though I was fairly active, I wasn't conscientious about any kind of regular fitness program.

I was working at a stressful desk job in health administration and, other than my avoidance of meat and fat, I was not doing anything that could be construed as prevention.

There is a strong history of type 2 diabetes in my family. As a physician, I should have realized that I was at increased risk and taken appropriate prevention measures. But, I didn't. In fact, I was clearly in denial because when I finally figured out that I had soaring blood sugars, I had already developed all the classic signs and symptoms. When that happened, it was my desire to simply buy some time to read up on diabetes therapy that led me to stop eating carbohydrates. I was aware that carbs drove blood sugar up and I wanted to minimize that while I basically figured out which drug to take.

My low-carb epiphany happened when I very quickly discovered that my blood sugars had corrected and that all my signs and symptoms had disappeared. I began losing about a pound a day and eventually lost over 30 lbs. My personal revelation that a low-carb diet was the magic bullet for my type 2 diabetes changed not only the trajectory of my personal health and well being but steered me onto a completely different career path. I began to study low-carb ketogenic diets and to meet the researchers and practitioners who were already familiar with its benefits. With the help of these colleagues, I was eventually able to conduct a dietary trial in a Canadian First Nations community where we put people on a modern interpretation of their traditional low-carb diet and followed them for a year. The benefits we observed in this study along with other individual case studies and the accumulating scientific literature in this area reinforced my conviction that this type of diet was far healthier than anything I had personally experienced or had been taught about during my medical education.

Nine years later, I am still eating a rigorously low-carb high-fat (LCHF) diet while maintaining excellent cardiometabolic markers without the need for any medications. My blood sugar tests are in the normal range and significantly better than the target values for type 2 diabetics indicated by the clinical treatment guidelines. Simply put, my previous full-blown type-2 diabetes remains in complete remission. My lipid profile is excellent while my inflammatory markers are in the basement. My last

CRP was 0.5 mg/L and my white blood cell count was 4.7 $10^9$/L. My waist has shrunk back from 36" to 31", not quite as slim as I was in my youth but close enough.

All this is great but perhaps the best part of this health transformation has been my exercise performance. I now find it easy to maintain a regular fitness schedule. I had always found it difficult to exercise very long in the past, which leads me to think that insulin resistance makes it hard to mobilize energy. The correction of my insulin resistance, and possibly leptin resistance, by avoiding carbs made it easy for me to work-out. Most days I do 30 minutes of cardio on a stationary bike and then sit-ups to exhaustion. I find this keeps me alert and energized throughout the day. It also strengthens my legs and core enough to do what I love most, you guessed it - downhill skiing.

We are fortunate in that we live only an hour's drive from Whistler, arguably the best ski resort in North America. When my son reached the age of three and we started him on skis, both my wife and I switched back to skis ourselves so that we could better manage him. We began to spend all our winter weekends there. And this is where my pre-low-carb and post-low-carb performance became most noticeably different. In my past life, although I loved the thrill of speed, I had little endurance. I rarely skied a full run nonstop, although the runs at Whistler Blackcomb are admittedly long.

As a low-carb skier I found my stamina had increased enormously. I started to ski all my favorite runs non-stop and, as my speed increased, I started skiing them with minimal turning. When I could do that on all the major runs on the mountain, I started doing the ultimate run, the seven kilometer long Peak-to-Creek that descends a full vertical mile from the very top to the very bottom of the mountain, non-stop. I would ski hard all day and then do the Peak-to-Creek as my last run. I would go flat out and, in the years I have been doing this, nobody has ever passed me. This may be because they don't know we are racing but I suspect it might be true even if they did. I know none of my ski buddies can do it. I also know that I could never have done it in my pre-low-carb days.

The other notable thing is my lack of hunger. On a ski day I will typically eat a big breakfast of steak, eggs and tomatoes or maybe a wedge of frittata with bacon and tomato with mayo. This is usually enough for me to ski all day. I might snack at lunch on a piece of cheese and pepperoni or sometimes I will eat a hamburger patty. Actually, the only reason I usually stop for lunch is because the people I ski with need to eat. I could forgo lunch and ski non-stop all day if I were on my own.

I always thought I was fast but I never actually timed myself. Last year, for Christmas, my wife gave me a little camera that attaches to my helmet. This year I recorded a descent and was somewhat amazed to discover that I did the 7 km in 6 minutes. That's an average speed of 70 kph (43 mph). Not bad for an old type 2 diabetic who is not an athlete or even a gym rat (I have posted that run on YouTube: www.tinyurl.com/myskirun).

Now, the only remaining thing that can possibly slow me down is my daughter Isabelle. Our son Alex is, at eleven, an accomplished skier. He and I ski the most difficult runs together. He did not inherit his father's "need-for-speed" gene, however. He is content with tree-skiing and other off-piste adventures and has recently taken up snow-boarding. Isabelle, on the other hand, may be a fellow speedster.

The product of a LCHF gestation, Isabelle was breastfed while my wife continued to avoid carbs. When Isabelle started eating solid foods, we prepared a medley of LCHF baby foods for her. She thrived on her meat sauces and pureed veggies with cheese and butter. Fairly quickly, she progressed to eating the foods we eat. Now, at the age of 2-1/2, when I barbeque a steak, I have to make an extra portion for her. She loves meat and insists on having red wine with it. Of course, all she gets is a small sip but, if we would let her, I think she would down the whole glass. She loves all kinds of foods ranging from olives to French cheeses to smoked salmon and all kinds of meats.

Being about average weight and height at birth, she shot up the growth curve and by her first birthday she had hit the 90th percentile for height and 70th for weight. She has that inner intensity and drive that will serve her well in whatever she chooses to do in life. Since she worships her older brother and wants to do everything he does, we started her skiing quite early. She became familiar with the upper slopes on Whistler Mountain at the age of 17 months. During the following summer, she would frequently ask to go skiing again and would often put on her ski boots to clomp around the house.

As the new season got underway, at the age of 28 months, she was skiing full runs with me trailing behind holding onto a tether to ensure she didn't get away. In just a few days of skiing her strength, coordination and stamina improved to the point where she can ski four full non-stop runs before taking a break. She can handle any slope and speed that I allow. So far, she has advanced to skiing the men's Olympic downhill race course which is ranked at the black diamond level of difficulty. If she falls, she quickly shakes it off and gets back on her feet. It is rare to see a child skiing the big runs at Whistler at such a young age. I think her LCHF baby diet gives her the amazing strength and stamina to do that at her tender age just as it does for me in my advanced years. She loves skiing. I am looking forward to that day in the future when she and I race down Peak-to-Creek non-stop. If she sticks to her LCHF diet, I have a feeling that day won't be too far off.

You can see Issy's first run on the downhill race course here: www.tinyurl. com/issyskiswhistler.

## David Dreyfuss -- Observations of an Older Low-Carb Recreational Athlete

Much of the focus of measuring athletic performance and the effects of various training and nutritional protocols is typically on young, mostly male, elite athletes with the goal of making the next world champion. You can get funding to help boost national pride by developing winners; it's much more difficult to promote general health with a program that doesn't have a high-value-add product to sell. But most of us have no ambitions (or talent) to reach elite performance levels. Nevertheless, exercise is widely accepted (by people of all nutritional persuasions) as part of a "healthy lifestyle," whether or not you have any competitive ambitions. And, of course, even among those who have at least some competitive ambitions, they are really only competing against a smaller group of "peers" (for example, the same gender and age group in the same city, or even just their own prior performance in similar events). So how does low-carb nutrition fit in? Very well, thank you! This is the story of one person's experience over several years. It's largely anecdotal, of course, but there are an ever growing number of similar anecdotes out there, and research (and books like this one that are based on that research) is slowly catching up with the anecdotes.

First, a bit of background. I am male, Caucasian, American-born and raised, age 56, 6 ft tall, ~185 lb (average for 2011). I am also a trained scientist and engineer; I am *not* an MD or a nutritional scientist).

Like a lot of American males, I was reasonably weight-stable in younger years with a tendency to overeat somewhat, which I could generally get away with, gaining only a couple of inches around the middle. As a college athlete (competitive fencer), my weight was about 165 lb; when not training, it tended to creep up to about 172 lb. As I got older, my weight remained generally stable, but followed the typical carb-fed American male pattern of a gain of about 1 lb per year up to about age 50. I then started to gain weight somewhat faster and to develop many of the typical symptoms referred to as "Metabolic Syndrome": weight gain, waist circumference gain, high blood pressure, high triglycerides, somewhat elevated fasting blood glucose. My weight topped out at about 220 lb.

About that time, I discovered Gary Taubes' book, which I found fascinating as an indictment of decades of terrible science and bad public policy. But it also prompted me to reconsider my own diet, and I adopted a low-carb lifestyle. I'm now four years in, and I've never looked back. My weight over those four years is shown in the Figure. You can spin the data in a variety of ways, but for the present purposes, I think a simple description is good enough. There was a "weight loss" phase of about eight months. Thereafter, I have been basically weight stable with a continued drift of about two pounds per year and a range of about ± 5 lb dominated by seasonal gain in the winter months and loss in the summer months. While some weight fluctuation may be attributable to "body recomposition" (muscle mass), I am, at this point, mostly an endurance athlete, and physical measurements (chest, waist, hips, thighs, calves, etc.) have not varied much. For most purposes, I can be considered "weight stable" for the last 3+ years. As has been observed by many adopters of the low-carb lifestyle, my metabolic syndrome symptoms have largely abated, though I still take a low-dose ACE-inhibitor for blood pressure control. I have had no reason to visit a doctor in that time for illness or injury. At present, I also supplement with Vitamin D, fish oil, and low-dose aspirin (and nothing else).

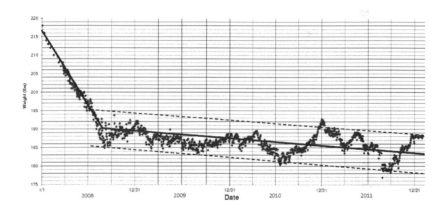

Throughout my life, I continued to be moderately if somewhat irregularly active mostly in non-competitive sports including hiking, biking, paddling, swimming, etc. When I did occasionally compete in something, I would typically finish in the middle of the pack somewhere at about twice the time of a world champion in the event. Other than the metabolic syndrome issues, my health has remained good, and I have no limiting injuries. My athletic focus has recently been on long-distance running, particularly trail running, and usually at a pace that is well within my aerobic limits. Typical runs are an hour or two, and weekly mileage has been typically around 30–40, but I occasionally run all day (8–12 hours), and I've run marathons and ultra-marathons up to 50 miles.

My transition from high-carb athletics to low-carb athletics coincided with my weight loss phase, so it's a little difficult to definitively separate out the effects of the weight loss from the effects of diet change. I also followed a rather different "induction" phase than that recommended by, for example, the Atkins Diet. I gradually reduced the carbs in my diet rather than going "cold turkey" and then backing off. As I got accustomed to leaving certain foods out of my diet, I no longer missed them. Regardless, of how I got there, I still felt the frequently-reported malaise during the first three weeks or so as my body adapted to fat-burning. After that, the problem was gone, and my "energy level" was much more consistent and stable both from day to day and from hour to hour during continuous exercise.

As a high-carb athlete, I used to "run out of fuel" (feel ravenously hungry and weak, probably with plunging blood sugar, though I never measured it) after about two hours of hard exercise. The effect could be blunted and pushed out somewhat with enough fiber, but it was always there. Long runs, paddles, or bike rides required regular refueling. I tended to gravitate toward more complex carbs, mostly because they seemed to "last longer." Simple sugars could give a short-term boost, but I got hungry again very quickly.

One of the things that I immediately noticed after switching to low-carb eating and getting through the transition period was that these extreme highs and lows just disappeared. In the same way that low-carb diets help people lose weight by eliminating the gnawing hunger that a post-carb crash creates, I just didn't need to eat frequently anymore. It still took me a long time to fully understand and take advantage. At first, I just assumed that I should still consume carbs during (and immediately after) a long bout of exercise. Just as with my general diet transition, I found myself gradually weaning my body from old habits. I was never particularly into "carb loading" (eating a high carb meal *before* endurance exercise), partly because, at that point, I had never done anything seriously long and competitive. I'd done very long days, but with generous stops for rest and food. Shortly after my weight loss phase is when I entered my first formal long event (a 50K trail race). I got through it, estimating that I had burned more calories than I had consumed, but I did consume carbs at every opportunity. (Most aid stations are stocked with hardly anything but carbs!) Of course, I "knew" about bonking, and I just assumed that it still applied to me, and that I would still run out of energy after two to three hours when my stored glycogen ran out.

The next step was to wonder whether the carbs were really necessary. Since I fueled my daily life with mostly fat, could I do the same for extended aerobic exercise? This too, I tried with gradually more strict application. First, I tried carrying a milk-based protein shake. It worked fine, but was it the carbs from the milk sugars that kept me going? Then I switched to coconut milk (with some added whey protein and flavorings, first "sweet" [Splenda and cocoa], then savory [chicken broth]). Coconut milk has very low sugar content. Total calories were still fairly generous: I would typically have a breakfast of a two-egg and cheese omelet plus bacon a couple of hours before starting, then take a few swallows of the coconut milk mixture every half hour or so starting after about two and a half hours. I continued this regimen during most long days for a year or so. It worked well. I had sustained energy all day and no stomach issues. Other than the inconvenience of having to carry all of my own food and ignoring the aid stations (if present) for anything other than water, I was happy. One water bottle could carry enough to last me for at least six to eight hours if I rationed it carefully.

More recently, I was prompted to look at the "science" behind "bonking," and generally found that the available hard data was pretty limited and inconclusive. Two "facts" are clear enough to stand up to scrutiny: (1) the body has much more limited stores of carbohydrates than fats that can be mobilized to fuel activity (see page 10), (2) there is generally a crossover that occurs with increasing level of effort (percentage of $VO_2Max$) from fat-fueling to carb-fueling. But, of course, the devil is in the details. Exactly where does the crossover occur? Can you influence it by training or nutrition? Traditional bonking lore tends to oversimplify the details and ignore variability. It appears that the crossover can, in fact, be influenced both by training (typically, by extended training below the crossover point—the "Maffetone" training method for runners, for example), and by nutrition. So it would seem to be a reasonable hypothesis that keto-adapted athletes don't bonk, or at least don't bonk as easily. This was a hypothesis that I could easily test on myself. Over the last year or so, I've run two street marathons, a trail marathon, and four trail ultra-marathons carrying no food and consuming only water. Total times ranged from about 4:20 to 9 hours. Bear in mind that I am not, and never have been, a speedy runner (best mile time ~6:30 at age 18, 6:45 at age 55). Conditions and levels of effort varied widely: some days I was running as hard as I could, others I was pacing someone slower or intentionally running slowly; some days were cool, some were hot; some routes were flat, some were hilly (thousands of feet of climb). But I never came close to bonking.

For all of these recent events, I started the day with a good low-carb breakfast, but then typically had little or no food until about 12 hours later, and consumed only water during the exercise. (In hot weather, I did take some salt, but I do not even use salt in cool weather.) I now hypothesize that even the breakfast is optional! When you use fat for fuel, the timing of meals is completely non-critical; you've got plenty on reserve at all times (a useful survival trait if you have to hunt on an empty stomach).

All the marketing hype about exactly what type of food you *must* consume at particular hours before, during, and after various sorts of exercise has thus become irrelevant for me. I still like to consume a little extra protein sometime in the 12 hours or so after strenuous exercise, but even the timing of that seems to be very flexible. I run when I want to for as long as I want to and eat when I get around to it. On a day-long expedition, I do get a little hungry around my normal lunchtime, but that fades quickly enough when I don't eat. (My normal eating habits are to eat three regular meals, so skipping a meal is an unusual event.)

Bonking is most commonly experienced in race situations where, for example, a marathon runner is pacing himself as fast as he can—probably at or near his aerobic limit. Some authors argue that if one stays below some limiting speed, one can replenish carbs fast enough to avoid bonking. Perhaps that could account for my ability to run 9+ hours at moderate speed without bonking. I have, however, also run a couple of street marathons at pretty close to my aerobic limit (heart rate increasing from 150 slowly to 160 through the race), and I experienced no bonking then either. Again, one could argue that I just can't run that far fast enough, but the experience is certainly suggestive that bonking can be avoided entirely by keto-adaptation.

So what's the gotcha? There has to be something wrong here. We've been pumping athletes full of carbs for decades now. So far, I haven't found any gotchas. As Dr. Phinney demonstrated (see page 22), there is no loss of peak performance. There seem to be real benefits for extended aerobic performance. Is it possible that some carb supplementation can give you a race performance boost? Maybe. Certainly you will find low-carb advocates who recommend such hybrid approaches. But I haven't seen any convincing data that suggests that any benefit is more than a placebo effect. I've experienced the effect myself: if you're really pushing, anything that can give you a temporary psychological boost can help. Everyone is familiar with the ability of most athletes to put on a finish-line sprint when they should be running on empty. Cheering spectators often boost performance. And some effects can be psycho-physical. For example, several studies have noted that performance can be improved just from swishing a sweet drink in the mouth and spitting it out.

If you've read the rest of this book, you've learned about the reduced inflammation and reduced oxidative damage that appears to go along with fat-burning instead of carb-burning. This can be difficult to measure rigorously, at least for the casual scientist/athlete with limited access to lab tests. However, I can certainly confirm anecdotally a subjective impression that the conclusions are correct. Even when completing my more extreme water-only runs, I experience much less post-event aches and pains and much faster recovery than I was accustomed to in the past. Of course, one can always attribute some of that experience to being generally better trained and stronger relative to the needs of the event, but I'm pretty sure that there's more to it than that. I can now do stuff that would have left me relatively crippled for a few days in the past and be ready to go out and do more the next day. I don't come anywhere close to wanting to just collapse at the finish. The muscles still work, and I can still use them fairly normally after a cool-down period. I don't detect any loss of strength, and I can perform similar resistance exercises as well the day after as I could the day before.

Dr. Phinney believes that increased sodium intake may be necessary during a low carb diet. My own experience has been that I can pretty much ignore the issue. I grew up in a low-salt household and still use added salt very sparingly. Outside of exercise and in cool weather, I use no electrolyte supplements. In very hot weather, I have a simple trick which seems to reduce my need for salt replacement: about half the water I use is dumped directly on my clothes. It's a lot more efficient to use it directly for evaporative cooling than to consume it and then sweat it out again. I follow the usual guidelines of drinking to thirst. I also generally keep track of urine output (i.e., that there is some every few hours) to double check that I'm not dehydrating excessively. Surprisingly, I've generally found that my total water consumption (again, anecdotally and not quantitatively) is significantly less now than it used to be. Just training? Nutrition? I don't know. I have no cramping and no stomach issues. As long as my muscles have adequate reserves, I just don't experience any problems.

In summary, then this is why I am and plan to remain a low-carb athlete:

1. I can easily remain weight stable.
2. I breathe slower when exercising (see page 35).
3. I don't need to eat even during long exercise.
4. I need less water during long exercise.
5. I recover faster and have less post-exercise pain.
6. My performance is equal to or better than when carb-fueled.
7. My general health is better.
8. I can exercise for several hours at a high level of effort without bonking.

Why would I even consider going back?

# REFERENCES

1. Volek JS, Phinney SD: The Art and Science of Low Carbohydrate Living: Beyond Obesity; May 2011.

2. Diamond J: The Worst Mistake in the History of the Human Race. *Discover Magazine* May 1987:64-66.

3. Catlin G: Letters and Notes on the Manners, Customs, and Conditions of North American Indians, vol. 1 and 2: reprinted Dover Pubs, NY,. 1971; 1844.

4. Jensen MD, Caruso M, Heiling V, Miles JM: Insulin regulation of lipolysis in nondiabetic and IDDM subjects. *Diabetes* 1989, 38(12):1595-1601.

5. Achten J, Gleeson M, Jeukendrup AE: Determination of the exercise intensity that elicits maximal fat oxidation. *Med Sci Sports Exerc* 2002, 34(1):92-97.

6. Phinney SD, Bistrian BR, Evans WJ, Gervino E, Blackburn GL: The human metabolic response to chronic ketosis without caloric restriction: preservation of submaximal exercise capability with reduced carbohydrate oxidation. *Metabolism* 1983, 32(8):769-776.

7. Phinney SD, Horton ES, Sims EA, Hanson JS, Danforth E, Jr., LaGrange BM: Capacity for moderate exercise in obese subjects after adaptation to a hypocaloric, ketogenic diet. *J Clin Invest* 1980, 66(5):1152-1161.

8.      Goedecke JH, St Clair Gibson A, Grobler L, Collins M, Noakes TD, Lambert EV: Determinants of the variability in respiratory exchange ratio at rest and during exercise in trained athletes. *Am J Physiol Endocrinol Metab* 2000, 279(6):E1325-1334.

9.      Venables MC, Achten J, Jeukendrup AE: Determinants of fat oxidation during exercise in healthy men and women: a cross-sectional study. *J Appl Physiol* 2005, 98(1):160-167.

10.     Hanson RW, Hakimi P: Born to run; the story of the PEPCK-Cmus mouse. *Biochimie* 2008, 90(6):838-842.

11.     McKenzie E, Holbrook T, Williamson K, Royer C, Valberg S, Hinchcliff K, Jose-Cunilleras E, Nelson S, Willard M, Davis M: Recovery of muscle glycogen concentrations in sled dogs during prolonged exercise. *Med Sci Sports Exerc* 2005, 37(8):1307-1312.

12.     McKenzie EC, Hinchcliff KW, Valberg SJ, Williamson KK, Payton ME, Davis MS: Assessment of alterations in triglyceride and glycogen concentrations in muscle tissue of Alaskan sled dogs during repetitive prolonged exercise. *Am J Vet Res* 2008, 69(8):1097-1103.

13.     VanItallie TB, Nufert TH: Ketones: metabolism's ugly duckling. *Nutr Rev* 2003, 61(10):327-341.

14.     Phinney SD, Bistrian BR, Wolfe RR, Blackburn GL: The human metabolic response to chronic ketosis without caloric restriction: physical and biochemical adaptation. *Metabolism* 1983, 32(8):757-768.

15.     Simi B, Sempore B, Mayet MH, Favier RJ: Additive effects of training and high-fat diet on energy metabolism during exercise. *J Appl Physiol* 1991, 71(1):197-203.

16.    Lambert EV, Speechly DP, Dennis SC, Noakes TD: Enhanced endurance in trained cyclists during moderate intensity exercise following 2 weeks adaptation to a high fat diet. *Eur J Appl Physiol Occup Physiol* 1994, 69(4):287-293.

17.    Volek JS, Quann EE, Forsythe CE: Low carbohydrate diets promote a more favorable body composition than low fat diets. . *Strength and Conditioning Journal* 2010, 32(1):42-47.

18.    Leino RL, Gerhart DZ, Duelli R, Enerson BE, Drewes LR: Diet-induced ketosis increases monocarboxylate transporter (MCT1) levels in rat brain. *Neurochem Int* 2001, 38(6):519-527.

19.    Nehlig A: Brain uptake and metabolism of ketone bodies in animal models. *Prostaglandins Leukot Essent Fatty Acids* 2004, 70(3):265-275.

20.    Cahill GF, Jr., Aoki TT: Alternate fuel utilization by brain. In: Cerebral Metabolism and Neural Function. Passonneau JV, et al, Eds. Williams & Wilkins, Baltimore, 1980. pp 234-42.

21.    Borkman M, Storlien LH, Pan DA, Jenkins AB, Chisholm DJ, Campbell LV: The relation between insulin sensitivity and the fatty-acid composition of skeletal-muscle phospholipids. *N Engl J Med* 1993, 328(4):238-244.

22.    Clore JN, Li J, Gill R, Gupta S, Spencer R, Azzam A, Zuelzer W, Rizzo WB, Blackard WG: Skeletal muscle phosphatidylcholine fatty acids and insulin sensitivity in normal humans. *Am J Physiol* 1998, 275(4 Pt 1):E665-670.

23.    Forsythe CE, Phinney SD, Fernandez ML, Quann EE, Wood RJ, Bibus DM, Kraemer WJ, Feinman RD, Volek JS: Comparison of low fat and low carbohydrate diets on circulating fatty acid composition and markers of inflammation. *Lipids* 2008, 43(1):65-77.

24. Sherwin RS, Hendler RG, Felig P: Effect of ketone infusions on amino acid and nitrogen metabolism in man. *J Clin Invest* 1975, 55(6):1382-1390.

25. Palaiologos G, Felig P: Effects of ketone bodies on amino acid metabolism in isolated rat diaphragm. *Biochem J* 1976, 154(3):709-716.

26. Young CM, Scanlan SS, Im HS, Lutwak L: Effect of body composition and other parameters in obese young men of carbohydrate level of reduction diet. *Am J Clin Nutr* 1971, 24(3):290-296.

27. Newsholme EA, Blomstrand E: Branched-chain amino acids and central fatigue. *J Nutr* 2006, 136(1 Suppl):274S-276S.

28. Bouchard C, Tremblay A, Despres JP, Theriault G, Nadeau A, Lupien PJ, Moorjani S, Prudhomme D, Fournier G: The response to exercise with constant energy intake in identical twins. *Obes Res* 1994, 2(5):400-410.

29. Heymsfield SB, Casper K, Hearn J, Guy D: Rate of weight loss during underfeeding: relation to level of physical activity. *Metabolism* 1989, 38(3):215-223.

30. Phinney SD, LaGrange BM, O'Connell M, Danforth E, Jr.: Effects of aerobic exercise on energy expenditure and nitrogen balance during very low calorie dieting. *Metabolism* 1988, 37(8):758-765.

31. Woo R, Garrow JS, Pi-Sunyer FX: Voluntary food intake during prolonged exercise in obese women. *Am J Clin Nutr* 1982, 36(3):478-484.

32. Kim do Y, Davis LM, Sullivan PG, Maalouf M, Simeone TA, van Brederode J, Rho JM: Ketone bodies are protective against oxidative stress in neocortical neurons. *J Neurochem* 2007, 101(5):1316-1326.

33.     Jarrett SG, Milder JB, Liang LP, Patel M: The ketogenic diet increases mitochondrial glutathione levels. *J Neurochem* 2008, 106(3):1044-1051.

34.     Sahlin K, Shabalina IG, Mattsson CM, Bakkman L, Fernstrom M, Rozhdestvenskaya Z, Enqvist JK, Nedergaard J, Ekblom B, Tonkonogi M: Ultraendurance exercise increases the production of reactive oxygen species in isolated mitochondria from human skeletal muscle. *J Appl Physiol* 2010, 108(4):780-787.

35.     Tuominen JA, Ebeling P, Bourey R, Koranyi L, Lamminen A, Rapola J, Sane T, Vuorinen-Markkola H, Koivisto VA: Postmarathon paradox: insulin resistance in the face of glycogen depletion. *Am J Physiol* 1996, 270(2 Pt 1):E336-343.

36.     Asp S, Rohde T, Richter EA: Impaired muscle glycogen resynthesis after a marathon is not caused by decreased muscle GLUT-4 content. *J Appl Physiol* 1997, 83(5):1482-1485.

37.     Himmelfarb J, Kane J, McMonagle E, Zaltas E, Bobzin S, Boddupalli S, Phinney S, Miller G: Alpha and gamma tocopherol metabolism in healthy subjects and patients with end-stage renal disease. *Kidney Int* 2003, 64(3):978-991.

38.     Jiang Q, Ames BN: Gamma-tocopherol, but not alpha-tocopherol, decreases proinflammatory eicosanoids and inflammation damage in rats. *Faseb J* 2003, 17(8):816-822.

39.     Amo K, Arai H, Uebanso T, Fukaya M, Koganei M, Sasaki H, Yamamoto H, Taketani Y, Takeda E: Effects of xylitol on metabolic parameters and visceral fat accumulation. *J Clin Biochem Nutr* 2011, 49(1):1-7.

40.     Long W, 3rd, Wells K, Englert V, Schmidt S, Hickey MS, Melby CL: Does prior acute exercise affect postexercise substrate oxidation in response to a high carbohydrate meal? *Nutr Metab (Lond)* 2008, 5:2.

41.     Holtz KA, Stephens BR, Sharoff CG, Chipkin SR, Braun B: The effect of carbohydrate availability following exercise on whole-body insulin action. *Appl Physiol Nutr Metab* 2008, 33(5):946-956.

42.     Stephens BR, Braun B: Impact of nutrient intake timing on the metabolic response to exercise. *Nutr Rev* 2008, 66(8):473-476.

43.     Bhattacharya K, Orton RC, Qi X, Mundy H, Morley DW, Champion MP, Eaton S, Tester RF, Lee PJ: A novel starch for the treatment of glycogen storage diseases. *J Inherit Metab Dis* 2007, 30(3):350-357.

44.     Correia CE, Bhattacharya K, Lee PJ, Shuster JJ, Theriaque DW, Shankar MN, Smit GP, Weinstein DA: Use of modified cornstarch therapy to extend fasting in glycogen storage disease types Ia and Ib. *Am J Clin Nutr* 2008, 88(5):1272-1276.

45.     Qi X, Band M, Tester R, Piggott J, Hurel SJ: Use of slow release starch (SRS) to treat hypoglycaemia in type 1 diabetics. *Nutrition & Food Science* 2010, 40(2):228-234.

46.     Roberts MD, Lockwood C, Dalbo VJ, Volek J, Kerksick CM: Ingestion of a high-molecular-weight hydrothermally modified waxy maize starch alters metabolic responses to prolonged exercise in trained cyclists. *Nutrition* 2010, 27:659-665.

47.     Rooyackers OE, Nair KS: Hormonal regulation of human muscle protein metabolism. *Annu Rev Nutr* 1997, 17:457-485.

48.     Staples AW, Burd NA, West DW, Currie KD, Atherton PJ, Moore DR, Rennie MJ, Macdonald MJ, Baker SK, Phillips SM: Carbohydrate Does Not Augment Exercise-Induced Protein Accretion versus Protein Alone. *Med Sci Sports Exerc* 2011, 43:1154-1161.

49.    Koopman R, Wagenmakers AJ, Manders RJ, Zorenc AH,
       Senden JM, Gorselink M, Keizer HA, van Loon LJ: Combined
       ingestion of protein and free leucine with carbohydrate
       increases postexercise muscle protein synthesis in vivo
       in male subjects. *Am J Physiol Endocrinol Metab* 2005,
       288(4):E645-653.

50.    Jakobsen MU, O'Reilly EJ, Heitmann BL, Pereira MA, Balter
       K, Fraser GE, Goldbourt U, Hallmans G, Knekt P, Liu S *et al*:
       Major types of dietary fat and risk of coronary heart disease:
       a pooled analysis of 11 cohort studies. *Am J Clin Nutr* 2009,
       89(5):1425-1432.

51.    Siri-Tarino PW, Sun Q, Hu FB, Krauss RM: Meta-analysis
       of prospective cohort studies evaluating the association of
       saturated fat with cardiovascular disease. *Am J Clin Nutr*
       2010, 91(3):535-546.

52.    Miettinen TA, Naukkarinen V, Huttunen JK, Mattila S, Kumlin
       T: Fatty-acid composition of serum lipids predicts myocardial
       infarction. *Br Med J (Clin Res Ed)* 1982, 285(6347):993-996.

53.    Simon JA, Hodgkins ML, Browner WS, Neuhaus JM, Bernert
       JT, Jr., Hulley SB: Serum fatty acids and the risk of coronary
       heart disease. *Am J Epidemiol* 1995, 142(5):469-476.

54.    Wang L, Folsom AR, Eckfeldt JH: Plasma fatty acid
       composition and incidence of coronary heart disease in middle
       aged adults: the Atherosclerosis Risk in Communities (ARIC)
       Study. *Nutr Metab Cardiovasc Dis* 2003, 13(5):256-266.

55.    Yamagishi K, Iso H, Yatsuya H, Tanabe N, Date C, Kikuchi
       S, Yamamoto A, Inaba Y, Tamakoshi A: Dietary intake of
       saturated fatty acids and mortality from cardiovascular
       disease in Japanese: the Japan Collaborative Cohort Study for
       Evaluation of Cancer Risk (JACC) Study. *Am J Clin Nutr* 2010,
       92(4):759-765.

56.    Patel PS, Sharp SJ, Jansen E, Luben RN, Khaw KT, Wareham NJ, Forouhi NG: Fatty acids measured in plasma and erythrocyte-membrane phospholipids and derived by food-frequency questionnaire and the risk of new-onset type 2 diabetes: a pilot study in the European Prospective Investigation into Cancer and Nutrition (EPIC)-Norfolk cohort. *Am J Clin Nutr* 2010, 92(5):1214-1222.

57.    Wang L, Folsom AR, Zheng ZJ, Pankow JS, Eckfeldt JH: Plasma fatty acid composition and incidence of diabetes in middle-aged adults: the Atherosclerosis Risk in Communities (ARIC) Study. *Am J Clin Nutr* 2003, 78(1):91-98.

58.    Warensjo E, Riserus U, Vessby B: Fatty acid composition of serum lipids predicts the development of the metabolic syndrome in men. *Diabetologia* 2005, 48(10):1999-2005.

59.    Forsythe CE, Phinney SD, Feinman RD, Volk BM, Freidenreich D, Quann E, Ballard K, Puglisi MJ, Maresh CM, Kraemer WJ *et al*: Limited effect of dietary saturated fat on plasma saturated fat in the context of a low carbohydrate diet. *Lipids* 2010, 45(10):947-962.

60.    Harris WS: Fish oil supplementation: evidence for health benefits. *Cleve Clin J Med* 2004, 71(3):208-210, 212, 215-208 passim.

61.    Kullo IJ, Khaleghi M, Hensrud DD: Markers of inflammation are inversely associated with VO$_2$ max in asymptomatic men. *J Appl Physiol* 2007, 102(4):1374-1379.

62.    Watkins BA, Hutchins H, Li Y, Seifert MF: The endocannabinoid signaling system: a marriage of PUFA and musculoskeletal health. *J Nutr Biochem* 2010, 21(12):1141-1152.

63.    Walser B, Giordano RM, Stebbins CL: Supplementation with omega-3 polyunsaturated fatty acids augments brachial artery dilation and blood flow during forearm contraction. *Eur J Appl Physiol* 2006, 97(3):347-354.

64.     Hill AM, Buckley JD, Murphy KJ, Howe PR: Combining fish-oil supplements with regular aerobic exercise improves body composition and cardiovascular disease risk factors. *Am J Clin Nutr* 2007, 85(5):1267-1274.

65.     Tartibian B, Maleki BH, Abbasi A: Omega-3 fatty acids supplementation attenuates inflammatory markers after eccentric exercise in untrained men. *Clin J Sport Med* 2011, 21(2):131-137.

66.     Nishiyama S, Irisa K, Matsubasa T, Higashi A, Matsuda I: Zinc status relates to hematological deficits in middle-aged women. *J Am Coll Nutr* 1998, 17(3):291-295.

67.     Nair KS, Welle SL, Halliday D, Campbell RG: Effect of beta-hydroxybutyrate on whole-body leucine kinetics and fractional mixed skeletal muscle protein synthesis in humans. *J Clin Invest* 1988, 82(1):198-205.

68.     Gilbert DL, Pyzik PL, Freeman JM: The ketogenic diet: seizure control correlates better with serum beta-hydroxybutyrate than with urine ketones. *J Child Neurol* 2000, 15(12):787-790.

69.     Musa-Veloso K, Likhodii SS, Cunnane SC: Breath acetone is a reliable indicator of ketosis in adults consuming ketogenic meals. *Am J Clin Nutr* 2002, 76(1):65-70.

70.     Koeslag JH, Levinrad LI, Lochner JD, Sive AA: Post-exercise ketosis in post-prandial exercise: effect of glucose and alanine ingestion in humans. *J Physiol* 1985, 358:395-403.

71.     Nosadini R, Datta H, Hodson A, Alberti KG: A possible mechanism for the anti-ketogenic action of alanine in the rat. *Biochem J* 1980, 190(2):323-332.

72.     Courtice FC, Douglas CG: The effect of prolonged muscular exercise on the metabolism. *Proc Roy Soc B* 1936, 119:381-439.

73.     Musa-Veloso K, Likhodii SS, Rarama E, Benoit S, Liu YM, Chartrand D, Curtis R, Carmant L, Lortie A, Comeau FJ *et al*: Breath acetone predicts plasma ketone bodies in children with epilepsy on a ketogenic diet. *Nutrition* 2006, 22(1):1-8.

74.     Kunesova M, Hainer V, Tvrzicka E, Phinney SD, Stich V, Parizkova J, Zak A, Stunkard AJ: Assessment of dietary and genetic factors influencing serum and adipose fatty acid composition in obese female identical twins. *Lipids* 2002, 37(1):27-32.

75.     King IB, Lemaitre RN, Kestin M: Effect of a low-fat diet on fatty acid composition in red cells, plasma phospholipids, and cholesterol esters: investigation of a biomarker of total fat intake. *Am J Clin Nutr* 2006, 83(2):227-236.

76.     Phinney SD, Kasim-Karakas S, Mueller W, Kunesova M: Palmitoleate: A Biomarker of Obesity and Potential Target for Treatment *Am J Clin Nutr* 2002, 75:373S.

77.     Raatz SK, Bibus D, Thomas W, Kris-Etherton P: Total fat intake modifies plasma fatty acid composition in humans. *J Nutr* 2001, 131(2):231-234.

# GLOSSARY

**AA** Arachidonic acid (aka arachidonate). A 20-carbon omega-6 essential fatty acid that provides vital physical properties to all cellular membranes, as well as serving as substrate for a myriad of oxylipids (eicosanoids) with hormonal and signaling functions. A common reductionist perspective labels AA as 'pro-inflammatory' and thus 'bad'. A more cosmopolitan view recognizes that AA is vital for many membrane functions (including insulin action), whereas it only can become 'pro-inflammatory' when released from membrane PL by specific phospholipase enzymes.

**AcAc** Aceto-acetate. One of two ketones produced from fatty acids by the liver. Usually converted to BOHB in muscle before being taken up and oxidized for energy by the brain.

**ATP** Adenosine tri-phosphate. This high energy phosphate is, along with creatine phosphate, the body's source of instant cellular energy. The release of one phosphorus produces adenosine di-phosphate (ADP), a free phosphorus molecule, and energy to power a host of functions including muscle contraction. Either glycolysis or oxidative phosphorylation can then re-attach a phosphorus to ADP, recreating the ATP energy charge.

**BCAA** Branched chain amino acids. These consist of leucine, iso-leucine, and valine. Chemically, these three amino acids can be regarded as short-chain fatty acids with an amino group attached. Once the amino group is detached (the first step in their breakdown), they can burned for energy in mitochondria like any other short-chain fatty acid such as pyruvate or BOHB.

**BMI**  Body mass index. This is calculated by dividing one's weight in kilograms by the square of one's height in meters. Values for adults between 18 and 25 are considered normal (aka healthy), 25-30 overweight, and above 30 is classified as obese. BMI is not a measure of body composition, but on average for large groups of subjects, BMI correlates well with body fat content. For individuals, however, BMI often correlates poorly with direct measures of adiposity, as for example in power athletes with expanded lean body mass.

**BOHB**  Beta-hydroxy butyrate. One of two ketones produced from fatty acids by the liver. The preferred ketone fuel to support the brain's energy needs.

**$CO_2$**  Carbon dioxide. Produced by the oxidative metabolism of glucose, fats, and amino acids. Its content in the blood is one of the two major drivers of respiration (along with blood oxygen content).

**CVD**  Cardiovascular disease. A combination of plaque formation in coronary vessel walls, plus hemorrhage into unstable plaques and thrombus (clot) formation that block blood flow to the heart muscle.

**DHA**  Docosahexaenoic acid. A 22-carbon omega-3 essential fatty acid found in human cell membranes, particularly in the central nervous system and the retina of the eye. Typically DHA is 10-fold more prevalent in human membranes than its metabolic precursor EPA (and 100-fold more so in the eye). Typically, the metabolic functions of DHA counter-balance those of AA, although in some membrane functions (such as insulin sensitivity) they are complementary.

**DRI**  Daily reference intake. This is a broad system used by the United States and Canada to develop recommendations for macronutrient and micronutrient intakes. It encompasses recommended dietary allowances (RDA), adequate intake (AI) and tolerable upper intake levels (UL). DRIs are relevant for healthcare policy and public health; they do not address individual circumstances and needs. Personal nutrient requirements may be higher or lower.

**DXA**   Duel energy x-ray absorptiometry (also called DEXA). Originally developed to accurately measure bone density, this technique is now available to measure body composition, including regional fat distribution. It uses a pair of x-ray beams of differing energies to measure tissue density. Because of the very narrow beams, the x-ray dose from this procedure is inconsequential compared to normal background radiation.

**EFA**   Essential fatty acid. These consist of two classes (omega-6 and omega-3) of 18- to 22-carbon polyunsaturates that serve both structural (membrane) and vitamin-like functions in humans.

**EPA**   Eicosapentaenoic acid. A 20-carbon omega-3 essential fatty acid. EPA represents about 50% of the omega-3 fatty acids found in most 'fish oil', but is typically between 1-10% of omega-3 fatty acids in human membranes. Because EPA directly antagonizes the pro-inflammatory effects of arachidonate, however, it is touted for its pharmacological properties. If this were true from a global perspective, however, most of the EPA we eat wouldn't be promptly converted to DHA. Go figure.

**HUFA**   Highly unsaturated fatty acids. This term refers to fatty acids of 20-carbon or longer chain length containing three or more double bonds. Most are from either the omega-6 or omega-3 classes, although the non-essential omega-9 biomarker of EFA deficiency (Mead acid – 20:3n-9) is also included in this classification.

**Kcal**   Kilocalorie, also referred to as 'Calorie'. A kilocalorie or Calorie (spelled with a capitol 'C') is approximately the amount of heat needed to raise the temperature of one liter of water by one degree Celsius. A 'calorie' is one one-thousandth this amount. While the use of the kilocalorie unit persists in North America, most of the rest of the world uses the SI unit 'joule' – there are 4.18 kilojoules (kJ) per kcal.

**LCT**   Long-chain triglycerides. Typical dietary fats in which the three individual fatty acids attached to the glycerol backbone have 14 or more carbons (and usually either 16 or 18 carbons). Absorption from the gut is via chylomicrons that enter the circulation via the lymphatics and the thoracic duct.

**MCT**    Medium-chain triglycerides.  Triglyceride molecules in which all or most of the fatty acids attached to the glycerol backbone have 8-12 carbons and no double bonds.  Absorption from the gut is followed by secretion into the portal vein and delivery to the liver, where most MCT are oxidized or made into ketones.

**MP-EFA**    Membrane phospholipid essential fatty acids.  Phospholipids have a polar end ('likes water') and a non-polar lipid end ('hates water').  When mixed in water, they align their non-polar ends, leaving the polar ends out towards the water.  This spontaneously generates the classic lipid bi-layer membrane structure upon which all cellular life depends.  Most phospholipid molecules have two fatty acids attached to the glycerol backbone.  Of these, one is usually a saturated fat and the other one a polyunsaturated fat of either the omega-6 or omega-3 class.

**MUFA**    Monounsaturated fatty acid.  A long-chain fatty acid containing one double bond.  In plant and mammalian metabolism, the predominant monounsaturate is the 18-carbon oleic acid (found in olive oil, high oleic safflower oil, lard, oolichan grease, and human adipose tissue).

**O$_2$**    Oxygen

**OFM**    Optimized Fat Metabolism is a ultra-endurance performance strategy developed by Peter Defty that integrates diet/fueling, training, rest/recovery, and lifestyle with the all-natural supplement, VESPA, to make a fundamental physiological shift to metabolizing fat as the primary and preferred aerobic energy source.  OFM challenges the conventional carbohydrate centric approach toward athletic performance and human health, using cutting edge nutritional and physiological science to help guide the program.  OFM does not completely eliminate carbohydrates, but makes "strategic" use of specific sources of carbohydrates before and during ultra-events.  Thus, while OFM is NOT necessarily a low-carb diet per se, many principles used in OFM are taken from research done on low-carbohydrate dietary regimens, including the concepts of nutritional ketosis and keto-adaptation.

**PEPCK**   Phosphoenolpyruvate carboxykinase. PEPCK is a key enzyme in gluconeogenesis (the pathway by which glucose is formed from non-carbohydrate sources). Fascinating work has shown that genetically modified animals that over-express this enzyme in skeletal muscle are leaner and more active.

**pH**   This is a measure of the concentration of free hydrogen in water. Pure water has a pH of about 7 (neutral). Values below 7 indicate acidity, and those above 7 indicate alkalinity. Technically, pH is the negative logarithm of the molar concentration of dissolved hydronium ions (H3O+).

**PL**   Phospholipid. A complex mix of amphloteric compounds that form into surfaces at lipid/water interfaces. Membranes contain a mix of PL, proteins, and free cholesterol. In human membranes, PL are typically enriched with HUFA relative to other fatty acid pools like adipose TG.

**PUFA**   Polyunsaturated fatty acid. Long-chain fatty acids that contain two or more double bonds. PUFAs carry a positive connotation because they have been shown to lower total serum cholesterol. Unfortunately it is lost on most observers that this occurs at the expense of HDL cholesterol (aka 'good' cholesterol), thus doing potentially as much harm as good. More PUFA (particularly HUFA) in membranes is good, but more PUFA in the diet (particularly in the context of a high fat diet) is more than likely bad. The major determinant of how much PUFA or HUFA you have in your membrane appears to be more a function of how slowly you destroy them rather than how much of them you eat.

**ROS**   Reactive oxygen species. Also called oxygen free radicals or free radicals. Typically oxygen-containing small molecules with a single free electron in the outer shell. These combine chemically with unsaturated fatty acids or proteins, and frequently create additional free radicals in a cascade-like reaction. This process is referred to as oxidative stress, and is countered by multiple enzymes and anti-oxidants that quench this reaction.

**RQ**   Respiratory quotient.   The ratio of the minute volumes of $CO_2$ produced divided by $O_2$ consumed ($VCO_2/VO_2$). Technically, this ratio uncorrected for protein metabolism is called the 'respiratory exchange ratio' (RER), however the two values are very similar and the terms tend to be used interchangeably. Glucose 'burns' in the body with an RQ of 1.0 and fat at 0.7. Ketogenesis (making more ketones that are being oxidized) reduces the RQ value, whereas lipogenesis raises it.

**SFA**  Saturated fatty acid.  This is a fascinating but much maligned category of fats.  In human tissue, these generally range from 14- to 22-carbons in length with no double bonds.  Lacking double bonds, saturated fats have higher melting points than unsaturated fats of comparable chain length – thus their tendency to be solid at room temperature (like butter, tallow, and lard).  The lack of double bonds also makes them far less prone to peroxidation (i.e., damage by oxygen free radicals) compared to monounsaturates and polyunsaturates,  imparting greater stability both within living tissue and as longer shelf-life of foods containing them.

**SOD**  Super oxide dismutase. A family of enzymes in and around mitochondria that quench (neutralize) reactive oxygen species.

**VO$_2$**  The volume of oxygen consumed per minute, whether at rest or during exercise.  This value can be expressed as total use by the whole body, or per kilogram of body weight.

**VO$_2$max**  The peak rate of oxygen consumed during a specific exercise. Typically this occurs as a plateau in oxygen consumption as exercise intensity is increased, and usually associated with an RQ (RER) value >1.0. In keto-adapted subjects, however, VO$_2$max is often reached at RQs less than 1 due to reduced anaerobic lactate production.  VO$_2$max can be expressed as a value for the individual as a whole (e.g., 3.5 liters per minute) or per kg of body weight (e.g., 50 ml/kg/min for a 70 kg individual).

# ABOUT THE AUTHORS

## JEFF VOLEK

I'm a dietitian-scientist, and dare I say author, who has spent 18 years studying diet and exercise effects on health and performance with a focus on low carbohydrate diets and dietary supplements. By way of credentials, I'm a registered dietitian (RD) thanks to training at Michigan State University and Penrose St Francis Hospital and I have a masters of science (MS) and doctor of philosophy (PhD) in Exercise Physiology from Happy Valley (Penn State).

Currently I profess in the Department of Kinesiology at the University of Connecticut. I'm fortunate to have colleagues smarter than me and a talented band of research fellows dedicated to shedding light on dark areas of nutrition. I've managed to author/co-author 200 and something scientific papers; a couple dozen of those from a series of heretical experiments showing positive responses to ketogenic diets. I also do a lot of research on dietary supplements (e.g., creatine, carnitine, whey protein, chromium) and resistance training.

I've been physically active my entire adolescent and adult life. I enjoyed competing in a range of sports in grade school eventually gravitating toward weightlifting in college. I was able to rekindle the thrill of competing in sports by training for powerlifting meets. I had marginal success winning a few local and state titles. I continue to go to the gym, although the frequency of my visits has decreased due to a demanding work schedule and two spirited boys who keep me on my toes. I do enjoy yard work. Thanks to residual benefits of powerlifting I derive satisfaction from shoveling the sometimes feet of snow in my rather long driveway, and moving half-ton (well maybe quarter ton) boulders into strategic locations around the house. Yes at least one of the authors of this booklet is a little warped.

## STEVE PHINNEY

The only form of superiority that I might have over Jeff is that I'm more warped than he. My interest in sports nutrition was kindled in medical school when I kept bonking when riding my bicycle over the mountains around San Francisco Bay. When I asked the sage professors at Stanford to help me diagnose my problem, their answer was, essentially "Get a car." So I abandoned California for a medical residency in Vermont, where I was told that bonking resulted from glycogen depletion and could be prevented by adequate dietary carbohydrate. So we did a study to prove that you can't exercise without a lot of dietary carbs, but we got the 'wrong' answer. Thus began my life as a heretic. We proved that given a few weeks of adaptation, endurance exercise was anything but impaired on a keto-genic diet. This convinced me that I needed to know much more about the basics of nutrition and metabolism, so I finished my medical training and went back to graduate school at MIT.

For 2 decades after my PhD at MIT, I held positions at the Universities of Vermont and Minnesota, and finally at UC Davis. As an academic physi-cian, my clinical practice included working with a few thousand patients following low carbohydrate weight loss diets. In addition to low carbo-hydrate diet research, my interests included the fatty acid composition of cell membranes and how diet affects inflammation and immunity. While my research was technically successful, it was a political disaster – I kept getting the 'wrong' answers. Eventually I got the message and moved into the more innovation-friendly biotechnology sector, and from there into independent consulting. In this position, I have both the time to write and the freedom to write what I want.

Besides cycling, I climb mountains, ski, cook for my hard-working wife and two epicurean teens, and maintain a year-around organic garden in California.